Death on the Menu

CJD
Victims
Diagnosis and Care

Families devastated by "Mad Cow"
Disease reveal their tragic stories

Harash Narang, FRCPath.
Newcastle upon Tyne
1997

Published by
H H Publishers
40 Brentwood Avenue
Newcastle upon Tyne NE2 3DH
England
Telephone: International: 44 191 2815311
Fax International: 44 191 2810611

&

Jodhpur Academic Publishers
G-139 Shastri Nagar
Jodhpur - 342003, India.
Telephone: International: 91 291 32139

UK. ISBN: 0- 97809530764 - 1 - 3

Acknowledgement

This book is dedicated to Brenda and Ken Bell for their unfailing support in troublous times and generous help without which the continuance of my work would have been frustrated and to my family and, in particular, my mother for her calmness and compassion for others which has been my inspiration. I would like my children, Anita and Anthony Narang to develop the same understanding for the feelings of others.

I would also like to acknowledge the support given to me by the relatives of CJD victim's and friends, especially Hazel Richardson who has helped me in many ways.

Harash K. Narang

"As I entered adult life, an air of optimism prevailed in medical circles. The main infections had been conquered. Polio, diphtheria and childhood diseases would disappear. TB was a minor illness. Life expectancy throughout western countries was rising rapidly.

Recently we have been faced, however, with more tragic news. Nature is goading us; new diseases have appeared. And in the case of one, "new variant" CJD, it may be that the carelessness of man in feeding his animals may have been a contributory factor.

This important book shows the misery + mayhem which has resulted + how it affects ordinary families. It should be compulsory reading".

Edward [illegible]

Foreword by

The Rt. Hon. Edwina Currie

As I entered adult life, an air of optimism prevailed in medical circles. The main infections had been conquered. Polio, diphtheria and childhood diseases would disappear. TB was a minor illness. Life expectancy throughout western countries was rising rapidly.

Recently we have been faced, however, with more tragic news. Nature is goading us; new diseases have appeared. And in the case of one, "new variant" CJD, it may be that the carelessness of man in feeding his animals may have been a contributory factor.

This important book shows the misery and mayhem which has resulted and how it affects ordinary families. It should be compulsory reading.

Edwina Currie
November, 1997

About the Author

Harash Narang, a Fellow of the Royal College of Pathologists and a scientist whose work and research is highly respected by many of his peers, is a long-time resident of Newcastle upon Tyne where he first examined the brain of a CJD victim and where, as a microbiologist, he dedicated himself to the investigation of the little-understood Transmissible Spongiform Encephalopathy diseases. The sudden emergence of BSE in the 1980s only served to strengthen his determination to pierce the veils of mystery surrounding its infectious agent.

His initial research into the diseases led him to the discovery of virus-like structures common in all brains infected with the disease, and ultimately to the development of a touch-method and urine test for its diagnosis in cattle and humans. His offer of details of these to The Ministry of Agriculture, Fisheries and Food in the UK at the start of the BSE epidemic was declined - at the probable cost of millions of pounds paid in compensation following the unnecessary slaughter of cattle mistakenly suspected of being infected.

The Authorities, at the beginning of the BSE epidemic, underestimated the gravity of the threat posed by that disease as they are now doing in their use of blood from CJD victims. Dr Narang's determination in the face of opposition to pursue his chosen field led to his being classed as a *persona non grata* and his job with the Public Health Service being terminated in 1994. Fortunately, through private funding from Mr. Ken Bell of Ken Bell International, he was able to continue his research.

Along with his laboratory work, Dr Narang has found time to meet with those most directly affected by the disease, the victims and their relatives and has heard their heart-rending accounts of their anguish and frustrations in providing care, sometimes in the face of an unsympathetic doctors.

In this book, in conversations with the author and in their own words, with only minimum editing leaving them somewhat disjointed, are the accounts of those who have lived alongside this most dreadful of fatal diseases for which there is, as yet, no treatment.

Dr. Narang would wish us all to bear in mind that:-

There, but for the grace of God, go each one of us.

Contents

Creutzfeldt-Jakob Disease

Never before has so much attention been given to the safety and nutritional value of the food we eat. And yet, looming ahead, brought about largely by the folly of some, we face what could become a scourge of biblical proportions, a disease introduced by man into cattle and then from cattle into man. That disease, Creutzfeldt-Jakob Disease (CJD), has transmitted through the food we have eaten. Now, equally, we face the lethal threat of its transmission through blood transfusions.

CJD was first recognised in 1921. It is attributed to a slow virus infection with an incubation period extending into many years. It is an inevitably fatal disease for which neither effective treatment nor cure has yet been found. In its classical form, it appears in the late middle-aged, those between 55 and 75 years. Death inevitably follows the appearance of the clinical symptoms, usually within six or seven months.

The incidence of classical CJD has been estimated to be some 1 case per 1,000,000 head of population worldwide. However, published data shows that the prevalence of CJD in different countries varies markedly. Annual incidence in some countries in ethnic groups may reach more than one per million, while in the general population in the USA it ranges from 0.4 to 0.26, France, 0.32, and in England 0.09. Since BSE appeared, the incidence in the UK has increased more than tenfold to one case per million. The extremely low incidence of CJD precluded the disease becoming known to the public until the outbreak of the BSE epidemic. From then on, it became a matter of growing concern to both the general public and the medical profession. In the past, few general medical practitioners (and, for that matter, few consultants) would have seen or come into contact with a single case throughout their whole career. It was a disease purely to be found in the neurology text books.

The change in public awareness came in the late 1980s with the shocking TV pictures of staggering cows. The knowledge that these cattle were to be our future food, and that they had been infected through the food they had eaten, made us question the safety of the beef sold in our shops. Public fear escalated when it became known that cooking was not sufficient to destroy the infective agent. The fear Mad Cow Disease caused radically changed our eating habits. Consumption of beef fell dramatically, (by some 25% at one stage): the Vegetarian Society was active and enjoyed unprecedented success in recruiting new members: more restaurants included vegetarian dishes on their menus and manufacturers introduced vegetarian brands.

The similarities between Mad Cow Disease and CJD were quickly and widely publicised. Both diseases showed similar clinical symptoms. Histopathological examination of brains from BSE and CJD cases showed the same damage in the brain cells, holes - vacuoles, in the medical terminology - giving rise to a sponge-like appearance under the microscope. The two diseases were obviously closely related. They are in fact both examples of Transmissible Spongiform Encephalopathy - TSE.

BSE had been caused by cattle eating infected foodstuff. Was it safe for humans to eat beef? Would they in turn be struck down with CJD? The official answer embodied in statements issued by or with the approval of MAFF failed to convince the public. Misinformation and confusion fuelled distrust.

From the smallest acorn, the mightiest Oak Tree grows! ... From the (almost) chance discovery of two or three cattle dying in Kent (England) in 1985 from a previously unknown disease sprang the biggest and costliest epidemic affecting animals ever experienced. Within a year of its first discovery, BSE had claimed the lives of more than 2,000 cattle in Great Britain. Deaths rose to 7,136 in 1989; 14,180 in 1990; 25,075 in 1991; 35,045 in 1992; 36,765 (or more) in 1993. The total figure, from the beginning of the epidemic up until August, 1994 was over 137,000 and has since risen to 177,000.

In 1986, when BSE made its first appearance, I was working for the Public Health Laboratory Service (PHLS), a body established to control the spread of infectious diseases under the direction of the Secretary of State. As a microbiologist, I had determined sixteen years earlier to study all that was known about the TSE agent and devote my research to adding to that knowledge in the hope that the more that was known, the more likely was the development of a treatment. But the PHLS did not accept that TSEs were obviously a crucially important part of their function. In a written report, dated 23 October 1990, Dr J.

W. G Smith, director of the PHLS Board, declared their official policy: "The PHLS position on slow virus work .. is that PHLS did not wish specifically to engage in this area at present, because it was being adequately addressed by other excellent research groups and there were many higher priorities for the limited research funds available to PHLS".

Realising the significance of the species-crossover of the agent from sheep to cattle and the threat it posed, not only to animals but also to the humans who ate them, everything my research had taught me prevented my agreeing with that policy and I maintained my interest.

Refusal to support this official policy and support the published statements of MAFF and Department of Health led to my being considered a "problem" by PHLS, being suspended for a long period and, finally, being made redundant. I was, however, able to continue my research, and worked closely with concerned families whose relatives had died.

"Beef is safe", MAFF said: and kept saying. The daughter of the Agriculture Minister, John Gummer, was paraded before the TV cameras with a burger in her hand.

"There is currently no scientific evidence that BSE can be transmitted to humans, or that eating beef causes CJD in humans. That issue is not in question. I am also advised that beef is a safe and wholesome product," said the Prime Minister, John Major.

Scientists who voiced their misgivings were labelled scaremongers. That was the official stance until 20th March, 1996 when, with his feet kicked from under him by emerging facts, Health Secretary Stephen Dorrell revealed the enormity of the Government's miscalculation. He admitted that ten young people had died with a previously unrecognised form of CJD.

Until forced to change by the emergence of scientific evidence to the contrary, the Authorities had remained steadfast in their confidence that the BSE infection posed no threat to man. In that, on the whole, they had support from the Southwood Committee Working Party.

The scientific community has been divided since the start of the epidemic as to whether this new disease, which had crossed the species barrier from sheep to cow, might jump again from cows to humans. The Government scientists who initially insisted that humans were safe are slowly changing their view, as if they had found some new evidence. But they were aware of the risk all the time. They were depending on the incubation periods being of such duration that disaster would not occur in infected people's life time. Some scientists have, in fact, changed their opinions and what, at one time, they saw as "No risk" they now see as a potential disaster. It must be stressed that these scientists have very little, if any, background knowledge of the subject and have never seen a CJD or BSE case. Nor have they worked with experimental animals. How could they be allowed and trusted to predict the outcome without any first-hand, working experience? In expressing their views, they have been gambling with human lives and the British economy.

Relationship of CJD to other neurological diseases

Before BSE and CJD surfaced, the general public was aware of some other common neurological diseases, such as Alzheimer's disease (AD) and multiple sclerosis (MS). With an aging population worldwide, some consider that there is the probability that AD will reach epidemic proportions in the twenty-first century. Those who have been unfortunate to have a relative develop this disease know the pain and suffering endured in caring for such cases.

The minimal incidence of CJD throughout the country and the general lack of first-hand experience by doctors combined with the similarities in symptoms the disease shared with other neurological diseases (for example, AD, etc.) has made diagnosis of the disease confusing. Undoubtedly, there have been many cases of wrong diagnosis, even in recent years when the link with BSE had heightened awareness of it. Such mis-diagnoses have provided little comfort or benefit for the families involved and the statements and policies of the Authorities have all too often contributed to the general feeling of worry and concern.

CJD is one of a number of neurological diseases. These include Huntington's Chorea, Pick's disease, MS and a number of other undiagnosed diseases. Unfortunately, especially in their initial clinical stages, many of these closely resemble Alzheimer's disease and therefore cannot always be distinguished in the living patient. CJD is extremely rare compared to

Alzheimer's which is at least 100 to 1,000 times more common and the difficulty is compounded by the large percentage of CJD patients presenting with dementia as a foremost feature thereby supporting a predilection towards a misdiagnosis of Alzheimer's.

Over and above the difficulty of differential diagnosis with AD, sufficient clinical blurring exists to mislead the doctor, especially in the earlier stages where the patient is having rapid, highly complex jerky movements. In these cases a diagnosis of Huntington's disease is often considered. This introduces another factor. Does the doctor tell the relatives of his unconfirmed suspicion of CJD or Huntington's disease? He is in a Catch - 22 situation. Avoiding offering any opinion risks losing their trust and confidence. On the other hand suspicion, which may later prove ungrounded, can generate a swell of fear and panic through the various branches of the families there and then. For the sake of relatives who consider they might be the next victims, the hereditary nature of Huntington's requires extra care by the consultant. The consequences of a mistaken diagnosis are illustrated in more than one of the cases which follow. The publicity given to CJD in recent years can leave few people with anything other than dread arising from that diagnosis. Whatever he elects to say or do - or even not say - carries a risk.

Equally difficult is the differentiation between CJD and the symptoms of a stroke. It is often the case that 5 to 10 per cent of CJD cases have been first diagnosed as stroke. The unique feature of CJD is that it alone of all human neurological diseases is transmissible. To confirm CJD, it is sometimes essential to transmit the disease experimentally.

It has also been found that, occasionally, CJD may be associated with other underlying diseases such as tumours, brain abscesses, AD, and strokes as demonstrated by transmission of the disease from these cases into animals. The difficulties faced in reaching the correct diagnosis may partially explain the low incidence of the disease. The current known cases perhaps represent only the tip of the iceberg. It is conceivable that large segments of the population are infected without any, or with only trivial or subclinical signs. The true nature of the incidence of the disease may, in fact, be concealed by some other co-existing disease.

The difficulty of diagnosis is further compounded by the lack of first-hand experience by most doctors (including specialists) in the past who have ended their careers without having come across a single case of CJD, and this lack of experience must obviously limit their ability to reach a reliable diagnosis in the face of such complexities. It may even be that the hospital where the patient has been admitted has no neurological facilities.

Relation between the family and medical staff

The physical and behavioural changes manifested by the patient are common to so many causes that these symptoms signify nothing unique for the clinician's guidance. No distinct clinical pattern is provided for diagnosis or treatment. Many patients show signs of memory loss or poor judgment, and many suffer depression and behave in a manner that indicates dementia - a treatable disorder. The duration of these symptoms also varies, therefore the final diagnosis must depend on experience, knowledge and the string of symptoms shown. Often, observations collected from the relatives form the only evidence the clinician has, though the medical profession is traditionally suspicious of what they hear from relatives. Relations between the family and staff can very easily become strained, argumentative and ill-natured and the ripple effect can sadly lead to a breakdown in trust.

The vital question which arises is: When should the relatives be told? Should they be alerted to the suspicion of CJD, should they be informed that the possibility of CJD is being investigated or should they be spared what might prove to be unnecessary worry and only told when final diagnosis is confirmed?

The decision of what to tell the relatives, and when, is one to be made by the clinician. Telling them too soon, before his suspicions are confirmed, can cause needless worry and anxiety. However, continual delays and references to further tests required can be seen as delaying tactics and cause greater distress when the final picture emerges. Uppermost in the doctor's mind must be the welfare of the patient under his or her care but he must also have consideration for the family. Confidence in the clinician is essential. The doctor cannot be seen to have made a wrong diagnosis. That is very difficult to "explain away". The whole area is a minefield.

Relatives who spoke to me all agreed they would rather have been told what the tests were being done for. Therefore, I feel relatives are entitled to be told what lies ahead and it is preferable that, unless there is good reason to the contrary, they be kept fully in the picture in all respects from the very beginning. If CJD is what is suspected, the relatives should be informed and offered full help to understand what this could involve in the same way as is done in the case of Huntington's, Alzheimer's disease and brain tumours.

Instances where the doctor has tried to delay or conceal the diagnosis have in the past been shown to cause greater anger and distress than would otherwise have arisen. The inevitable delays necessitated by testing and awaiting results are all causes of stress to the family and require full and candid explanation. The relatives must be made aware why the diagnosis is difficult and inevitably time-consuming but be reassured that all is being done to assuage their anxiety and that they are being given full details as and when these become available. Trust, confidence and an understanding between medical staff and family must be established and maintained. The family must realise that, in this field, progress can only be made through a process of elimination and that a series of working hypotheses is often essential.

CJD and the family

For the families, CJD is a profound calamity. Hardship, distress and suffering ends in inevitable tragedy. Growing awareness of the devastating nature of the disease, its course and its inevitable outcome must raise public and professional awareness and understanding of the anguish it causes in those who nurse and care for the victim. All too often, that understanding seems sadly lacking. Faced with a patient for whom there is no available treatment or hope of a cure, and with nothing to offer the immediate family by way of encouragement, the need for compassion and sympathy is obvious. There is nothing the consultant can say or do to sugar the pill. His diagnosis has robbed the family of all hope and, whether or not they understand all the implications, it has also condemned them to months of soul-destroying, round-the-clock care for a rapidly-declining loved one. The family's reaction to this horrifying diagnosis may range from initial incredulity, through blind acceptance and determination to make the best of things, to anger at the doctor for all the delays and uncertainties they have endured only to end up with a no-hope verdict, or anger at the system for leaving them unsupported in their time of need.

At present, very little consideration has been given to how CJD patients should be handled and helped. Very little advice has been provided and the carers, all too often, have been left, alone and unaided, to make do as best they can. There is also the question of whether there is a health risk to others from living alongside a CJD case, but no-one seems prepared to accept the responsibility for deciding what precautions should be observed. This is true whether the patient is at home or in an established institution. Decisions as to what should be done are taken on the spot. When the incidence of the disease was low, the reluctance of the central authorities to mount an Information & Education campaign could, perhaps, be understood - but not condoned - on grounds of cost per patient. It cannot be justified now.

Needful of care, attention, constant nursing and human comforting as the invalid will be, so too are those who are doomed to provide that all-too-often unappreciated attendance. Professional carers may be used to the difficulties: relatives, with the onus thrust on them, unexpectedly and with inadequate preparation, seldom are. Perhaps their need for help to give them the strength to face their daily struggles, frustrations and heart-rending worries is greater even than the patient's.

There is, at present, no recommended course for the care and treatment of CJD patients, and few guidelines to help those who are accepting the responsibility for their care on a full-time basis. hospitals, acknowledging their inability to provide treatment, are reluctant to commit their limited facilities on a continuing basis. Neither nursing homes nor hospices provide the answer in most cases, ruled out either by their reluctance to accept such patients or by cost.

For want of an acceptable alternative, home care is usually the only answer. The carer faces unceasing trials and frustrations. Undisturbed sleep becomes an unexpected treat. Household chores become increasingly irksome, with continual interruptions. Trips out to nearby shops become events, luxuries prized for their infrequency. Care requires round-the-clock, on-the-spot availability with no bright light at the end of the tunnel. Death is the inevitable outcome.

The stress on the carer, probably a spouse, child or parent, can be enormous, bringing frictions within the family and ruin to family relationships. Only those immediately and intimately involved can know the anguish that accompanies the disease. Starting from the uncertainty and unawareness of what lies ahead when first told that CJD has been diagnosed, through the devastating months of constantly seeing and living with a disintegrating loved one with no hope for any release, to the inevitable death. Can that death be seen as anything but a welcome release, devoutly to be looked forward to by all in the family, invalid and relatives alike?

Financial problems will, almost inevitably, arise. The household routines will be thrown into disarray, family relations may be stretched to breaking-point. The lot of any young children living at home must be horrendous. They have to deal with the scars and traumas left by thoughtless derisory references to "mad cows" and ostracism by classmates from fear of infection. And there is the ever-present anxiety. Am I next? Is this dreadful disease infectious? Is the infection already in me? If we both ate the same food, when will I start to show the signs?

The common reaction when the CJD virus strikes (or, perhaps more accurately, shows the symptoms of having struck) is: "Why me?", or "Why in our family?" With the sole exception of the so-called "Iatrogenic Cases" (the accidental transmission of the agent from an existing case to another individual as described in the following paragraph), there are no available answers to these questions. Susceptibility and vulnerability to the CJD virus remain among the many mysteries surrounding the disease.

Treatment

Modern medical science has done much to relieve the anguish and agony of diseases which, in the past, led inevitably to a slow and painful death. Some are now treatable inasmuch as their progress is halted or slowed; a few are now curable. To be treatable, however, the cause of the illness must be known and its diagnosis made at an early stage. Transmissible diseases can be prevented by understanding the mode of infection and pre-immunising potential hosts. There is, however, no treatment for CJD and, therefore, top priority must be given to identifying the agent. Only now, ten years too late, and after the expenditure of millions of pounds with little benefit to show, are the official scientists being given encouragement - and another million pounds - so that they can rush ahead and begin the research which should already have been completed.

Is Post-mortem Essential?

Under the prevailing official policy, although the patient is clinically diagnosed as suffering from CJD, CJD is not considered as the cause of the death until that diagnosis has been confirmed by brain examination. Such examination is not possible without a post-mortem and, as the law stands, for that the agreement of the relatives is required. The strain endured by these relatives over an extended period of months, and their natural desire to see things over and done with, often precludes their prolonging the agony by requesting and then waiting for the results of a post-mortem. They fail to appreciate its importance. Since a post-mortem is not mandatory, relatives do not realise its significance and consequently many CJD case are not included in the official count.

The policy of the Government in establishing the CJD Surveillance Unit, at great cost, to monitor changes in the incidence and pattern of the disease without, at the same time, providing the mechanism to ensure the accuracy of its data is hard to understand. For doctors merely to ask relatives - “You don’t want a post mortem, do you?” is just not enough. These doctors should be giving a positive lead. The importance of post-mortem should be stressed in simple words and it should be recommended to relatives. All too often, this has not happened in the past. With hindsight, many of the relatives regret not having agreed and feel that doctors should have explained the situation to them more fully. Relatives are united in believing that the disease should be made notifiable.

In some cases, a brain biopsy is done. There is, however, a particular problem in interpretation of biopsies in suspected CJD cases, and therefore biopsy in such cases is now discouraged.

The Official Response: Government Policy

At about the same time as BSE was coming to be publicly and widely known, another disease was also engaging widespread attention. That was AIDS. To control that disease the Government took measures to make the public aware of it and of how infection could be avoided. No such immediate steps were taken to safeguard against the threat raised by BSE. Since the first isolated BSE case appeared, a further 177,000 cases have been confirmed, many more animals were killed while asymptomatic and their meat sold for human consumption.

Now millions of cows are doomed to die because, in the absence of a test to identify which cows are infected, cattle over the age of 30 months are banned from the human or animal food chain. In the case of AIDS, neither Government nor industry had any interests at risk: on the contrary, pharmaceutical industries had gains to make. Large sums of money were spent on publicity and research. The BSE story is very different.

Uncertainty as to where and when the disease will next strike only serves to exacerbate the fear and anxiety it brings. Any vacillation and changing of policies to meet the fear only adds to it. That, too often, has been the case in this country - unlike the USA. In 1985, Dr. Mortimer Lipsett of the (US) National Institutes of Health was alerted to three unexpected deaths among young persons with pathology resembling CJD, the common factor being that they all had previously received growth hormone treatment. Within two weeks, paediatricians around the country has been advised to be on the lookout for unexplained neurological deaths. When, two months later, two more cases surfaced, that hormone treatment was immediately banned and withdrawn and all recipients of the treatment were informed.

The admission that CJD and BSE were linked erupted immediately through both home and continental markets bringing new regulations for the preparation of meat, new rules controlling what should be allowed for human consumption and, overseas, bans on the import of British beef. What it did not bring was comfort and succour for those struck down by the infection. The lack of compassionate and immediate action is unforgivable. Not even a Guidance for Carers pamphlet has so far been published by the Ministry who have, so often in the past, rushed out Guides to coping with all manner of health-related issues - smoking, AIDS, drugs & solvent abuse, to mention three. Marginalised by the government, CJD victims became pariahs. They were cold-shouldered by a Health Service which, unable to offer or provide help, seemed all too often, to begrudge even basic human comfort and compassion either to them or their carers. Even Funeral Directors are known to have asserted the need for special precautions: nine-foot deep burial and sealed coffins.

Over the last decade, attitudes have varied, ranging from the "remote risk" to a potential apocalyptic pandemic. The validity of the former is to be devoutly prayed for; the devastation of the latter, should it come to be realised, must be minimised by all means at our disposal.

The risk to humans is very real: as real as the threat to our cattle ten years ago. Errors of judgment then, influenced perhaps by financial and economic considerations, paved the way for disastrous policies that led to the deaths of a large number of cattle. These same policies, by allowing the human consumption of infected beef to continue, may have introduced into man one of the most deadly scourges in history. Neither politics nor economics should again be allowed to stand in the way of safe-guarding human health. Science alone may provide a defence or, at least, a means to lessen the damage. With that aim in mind, the attention of the best scientists in the world, drawing on their experience and knowledge of the disease, must be focused on the challenge and empowered to tell the politicians what must be done. Hard decisions may be required: costs may be high. So be it. Our health alone must be the paramount consideration. The first of these decisions are required now. The risk is known to be real: twenty-three people are already admitted to have died.

Top priority must be given to the identification and determination of the infective agent and its nature. Little can be achieved to defeat it without more knowledge. The start towards that must be made now. Equally important, such defensive measures as are advised, must be put in position without delay, and these, of necessity, require a simple means for the early detection of the infection.

Unlike the US policy of controlling the spread of disease, in the UK, both science and scientists were waylaid by a political agenda. The Government refused to acknowledge the BSE danger. The chief priority was to reassure domestic consumers and the world at large that British beef was safe to eat. The BSE threat was needlessly prolonged.

Government scientists maintain that the BSE strain of the agent has infected humans but is limited to the young. The tragic stories of relatives in this book reveal that all age groups are equally vulnerable to the BSE agent.

Epidemiological Surveys

Epidemiological studies have so far failed to reveal any natural mechanism to explain the transmission of the disease either in sporadic form or within families. This leaves many unanswered questions. The existence of vertical transmission in humans seems very unlikely, while environmental factors remain unexplored. Some of the evidence points to genetic factors playing a role in providing entry to infective agents, thus causing the clinical onset in a familial group which may be classified as "high risk".

Several studies have examined the hypothesis of a workplace link, particularly where health care professionals and workers with animals on farms are concerned. In these studies, no significant differences have been found between such employees and the general population. It must, of course, be remembered that the infection transmits within the tissues alone and that even regular contact with infected animals will pose no threat to health. Absorption of infected tissue is what creates the risk and, with a rare disease with incubation periods of 10 to 30 years or more, assessing the probability of such absorption is hard, if not impossible. It is easy to explain how workers on farms, in butchers' shops and abattoirs fall victim to the infection; not so easy to account for it in nuns, vicars and engineers. The meat-related group come into contact with animal tissue daily but, with the latter group such information is unavailable, and the patient is often too ill to supply it. In these situations, only third party accounts are available and, when we have difficulty remembering what we had to eat last week ourselves, such accounts have only limited value. What past studies have failed to include is activities and hobbies which may have provided the occasion for transmission of the agent into seemingly low-risk people. My studies, for the first time, reveal the possibility of such links.

I came across one patient who died of CJD. He was an engineer, but he regularly went to a local abattoir for animal heads which he would take home and split open with an axe to feed his dogs. In another case, it was a butcher's wife who died. She regularly helped him kill clinically affected animals in his backyard, and the meat was then sold to the public. In another case, heads were used for the preparation of soup.

Since animals inoculated with a single dose, do develop the clinical disease, it is obvious that one infective dose alone is enough to start the process. In animals where disease has developed following ingestion of food, transmission was so irregular that it remains open whether it was the gastrointestinal tract itself or areas of mucosal abrasions which provided the true portal that is the. way in. Why some get the disease and others do not is not as yet known. In some patients, the portal entry may be through bad teeth or ulcerations of the gums or lips. The disease is known to develop with a significantly shorter incubation time where there are ulcerations. The long incubation period of the disease may mean that some humans, even if infected, do not clinically develop the disease during their lifetime.

In experiments, it has been shown that feeding of scrapie-infected brains to mink does not produce clinical disease as BSE-infected brains would do and, therefore, it is possible that scrapie was either not transmitted to man through the food chain or else man has developed a natural immunity to it. However, it is possible that scrapie did transmit to the occasional man through cuts - direct inoculation - or through an intermediary host which, in the opinion of some researchers, may have been cats. This hypothesis explains the low incidence of CJD. Although BSE is relatively restricted in its geographic distribution compared with the worldwide distribution of meat and meat products, it is a matter of major worldwide concern and worry. The populations of Australia and New Zealand which are free from scrapie would, on this basis, be at greater risk than the native UK population if exposed to the BSE agent. In my opinion, it is more than possible that exposure first to the scrapie strain provides a form of protection which acts as a vaccine.

Atypical Clinical Symptoms of Narang Disease CJD

Following its identification in the 1920s, CJD was recognised as affecting predominantly the middle-aged and elderly, with only a few exceptions, chiefly the so-called "iatrogenic cases", where infection is transmitted accidentally during surgical procedures (as detailed in my book, "The Link").

During the course of my studies which I had begun in 1970, I found, for the first time, cases with novel features starting to appear from 1988. From then on, there was a significant increase in the number of such cases. These cases - where the patient had balancing difficulties as a leading symptom - formed a new category. Based on this criterion, they came to be classified by me as "atypical" cases. I also observed that brain pathology closely resembled that seen in BSE. In both these respects atypical CJD differed from the "classical" type. Some seven years later, in 1996, the CJD Surveillance Unit admitted having also identified CJD cases under the age of 40.

None of these new cases matched the established diagnostic criteria for typical CJD. What I had described as "atypical" strain, the Surveillance Unit preferred to call a "new variant strain" of CJD. The main difference between the "old classic" and "new" strain CJD is that the classic disease starts with dementia, while the new starts with balancing problems and difficulties in walking. Most of the known cases of this new form follow a set pattern: the initial psychological problems and depression, followed by physical instability, ataxia, coma and death. The duration of the illness can extend for months, unlike the weeks more common in sporadic, traditional cases. The relatives have often had difficulty persuading their doctors that there is something seriously wrong with the patient. In the past, however, a few cases of an ataxic-cerebellar form of CJD have been also reported. These cases had rapidly progressive disturbances of muscular control; involuntary rhythmic jerking movements, dementia, progressing to coma and, finally, a state of generalised muscular rigidity in which the involuntary movements tend to disappear. The duration of the disease in these cases was about 12 to 18 months; similar to that seen in atypical CJD. The name "new variant strain" is therefore misleading and therefore the name "Narang disease " was proposed.

Furthermore, a detailed study of the history of scrapie would suggest that this so-called "new variant" is, in fact, one of the old, rare strains of scrapie in sheep - the "trembling type" - which has been selected by the cattle and which is now commonly known as BSE.

Doctors from the CJD Surveillance Unit have told some families that their relative could not have had BSE strain because they were too old to be infected with it. What, in effect, they are saying is, if you are over 40 eat BSE infected cattle as much as you like, you won't get BSE. This is questionable. Experiments have demonstrated that the incubation period is reduced by increasing the host's age at the time of infection; and that the older the animal when infected, the shorter the incubation period.

It would appear that this new strain affects young and old alike. The clinical course it follows, however, differs from that usually seen in sporadic CJD. The initial diagnosis in all my cases was made by demonstrating nemavirus and SAF in their brains before the results of histopathological investigation were available (for details see "The Link"). In many of the cases, behavioural and mood changes along with depression were included in the symptoms and, as is apparent from case notes, their symptoms were so different from typical CJD cases as to merit them being referred to a psychiatrist. At the early stage balancing and walking had become difficult with the patient tending to trip and stumble. Memory impairment develops and becomes more apparent with the progression of disease and balancing and walking become increasingly difficult. Based on conventional and accepted diagnostic criteria for CJD, none of these cases would be even classified as "probable" cases of CJD on clinical grounds. None of them had the typical EEG patterns traditionally associated with CJD although, during the final stage, EEG results did show some slow amplitude activity.

When this form of the disease, so unlike the traditional strain in the early symptoms shown, appeared in young people under the age of 41, it caused alarm bells to ring. Urgent research and study was required.

The existence of a relationship between the BSE strain of the agent and CJD crossed my mind in 1988 and the likelihood of such a link had to be quickly tested and established. To do so, I started a series of experiments in 1989, inoculating brain tissue from "atypical" CJD cases into laboratory animals. Some 18 months later, but before the work could be completed, I was asked by Dr. Nigel Lightfoot, Director of the PHLS, Newcastle to destroy the test animals on the grounds of safety. Why such fundamental experiments to examine any possible link between BSE and CJD should have been terminated baffles me.

It is strange that such vital experiments for the early detection of a BSE and CJD link and the possible development of a vaccine to protect both cows and humans were terminated. Even now, some seven years later after MAFF officially acknowledged in March, 1996 that: "humans have been infected with a new variant of the scrapie agent and the most likely source is BSE infected meat", no one has questioned the decisions of Dr. Lightfoot and the PHLS and asked them to provide an explanation.

Inadvertent inoculation?

My view is that people who have eaten scrapie-infected sheep have, for some unexplained reason, acquired some degree of protection against BSE-strain CJD and, therefore, are less likely to catch BSE infection. That does not imply that such people can safely eat BSE-infected meat. The risk to them may be smaller, but I strongly believe that all age groups are at risk. No-one can estimate how many are still incubating the disease. Thirty years ago, lamb was eaten more often then beef. More recently, however, younger people have developed a greater taste for beef and this may explain why younger people appear to be at the greatest risk from BSE. Involuntarily and unintentionally, the British public are taking part in the first natural BSE animal-to-human transmission experiment and the final outcome is unpredictable. What goes without saying is that top priority must be given to the development of an anti-BSE vaccine both for humans and animals.

CJD and Blood Transfusion

CJD transmission is a risk which the Blood Transfusion Service fully know but there is little they can do to ensure the purity of the blood they daily collect and distribute. Since there is as yet no firm evidence in humans that the infective agent can transmit through blood, it is at present considered a low risk. It has been known from Japanese and American studies since 1980, and before BSE appeared, that mice inoculated with human blood from cases of CJD develop the disease, thus conclusively demonstrating the presence of the CJD agent in blood, regardless of the strain. Transmission studies in mice have shown that each millilitre of blood contains 1000 units of infectivity.

No blood or blood product from a CJD case can be regarded as infection-free: none must be used. As soon as the possibility is suspected that a blood donor may be suffering from CJD, as a precaution, the Blood Transfusion authorities must be notified. There is no margin of safety. All the Transfusion Service is doing in the attempt to minimise the risk is pursuing their policy of advising relatives of CJD victims and growth hormone recipients not to donate blood. The real risk is to the patient who receives a transfusion taken from an apparently healthy donor who, some few months later, dies from CJD.

What is known from one epidemiological study in the UK is that out of 202 definite and probable CJD cases, 21 had received a blood transfusion, and 29 had donated blood. The need for medical records being continually updated and such vital information being made available within the Health Service is obvious. The recent appearance of BSE-strain CJD and the increase in the number of cases, particularly in the blood-donor age group, highlight the need for accurate records to be available for future study. Several cases reported in this book were blood donors.

The official stance on blood transfusion is the same as it was for transmission of BSE to humans: the risk is "remote". But it is an established fact that blood from CJD cases is infectious for animals. Since human blood for human use does not involve a species barrier, infection is the more likely. The only way to remove this risk and reassure the public is to test all blood donors and there is no alternative but to do so. Many of the patients described later in this book were diagnosed by my urine test.

Identifying CJD

Sporadic CJD appears in patients who have previously enjoyed good health and it usually presents during middle and late life. It manifests in a wide variety of clinical symptoms including dementia. The first appearance of the symptoms is normally followed by a fairly rapid deterioration over a period of four to seven months during which the disease is almost invariably accompanied by a variety of neurological abnormalities, particularly visual, and cerebellar deficits, often in association with myoclonus and other involuntary movements. Some CJD patients develop typical clinical features. With our current state of knowledge, these cases should present no problems in clinical diagnosis. The presence of one of these clinical symptoms, however, does not mean that the patient presenting it will develop CJD. A whole string of symptoms observed in an orderly fashion is required and, even then, clinical diagnosis may be difficult.

Neither individuals nor their relatives who suspect they are suffering from CJD should attempt self-diagnosis and diagnose CJD as the trouble. They should and must seek medical help and advice. This book is not written as a "Beginners' Guide to Diagnosing CJD". It is hoped, however, that it will contribute to a better understanding of how the disease develops and how best the friends and relatives of the victim can cope and live with its catastrophic development.

CJD expresses itself in so many diverse ways that clinical diagnosis usually comes only after a history of seemingly unrelated problems occurring over a period of months and giving rise to concern only when something so bizarre occurs that other family members cannot explain it away. Peculiarities in behaviour, particularly if not extreme and occurring only occasionally, tend to be ignored both by the patient and relatives, or considered insignificant. It is true that, after diagnosis, care-givers and relatives can, with hindsight, often recall a number of events that were in fact warning signs. Some would say that retrospective data, of course, is not very trustworthy, particularly if obtained belatedly. It may indeed be too late to help the patient, but the greater the collection of comparative notes available to doctors, care givers and public alike, the greater the contribution to an understanding of the disease. This is what I have tried to do in this book.

Many patients exhibit non-specific symptoms common to other conditions which begin weeks or months before neurological signs. These symptoms usually consist of uncertainty, feelings of anxiety, disturbance in sleeping, changes in eating patterns and weight loss, with only minimal mental deterioration. In the great majority of patients, the onset of the illness has been reported to be rather gradual. The first sign of the illness has often been an episode of confusion, vertigo, diplopia, or blurred vision. Less often, a sense of clumsiness, tremor, slight paralysis, or an abnormal sensation in one limb were also observed. In patients with the more typical subacute onset, they reported a gradual failure of memory taking the form of an inability to remember names or recent events, losing one's way in familiar surroundings, or general confusion. Behavioural abnormalities usually resulted from an agitated or depressed state of mind. Defects in higher cortical function were often manifest, where the patient had difficulty in finding words, performing simple arithmetic or writing correctly. The patients were rarely aggressive and almost never violent.

Some patients have experienced only physical symptoms, others have suffered a mixture of both mental and physical symptoms. In some patients, the onset of neurological symptoms might be abrupt, with eyesight problems, the development of uncontrolled shaking, even paralysis as in a stroke-like presentation, followed by emotional deterioration and eventual dementing with severe loss of analytical capability. The symptoms also include gait disturbance, and a sensation of vertigo. However, the manifestation of any one or more of such symptoms does not necessarily mean the existence of CJD in the patient.

Clinical Stages of CJD

The clinical course of the neurological syndrome can in the majority of cases be divided into three stages:-

The First Stage of the Classical CJD is a developmental stage in which symptoms begin to build up over several weeks. These include tiredness, physical discomfort, odd and painful sensations in the limbs which often present at the onset but are never conspicuous. Apart from these general complaints, mild apprehension, fatigue, morbid anxiety about one's health (hypochondria), inability to concentrate and forgetfulness are also observed. Other presenting symptoms include weakness or loss of control of a limb with a lack of coordination of movement, failure to arrange words in their proper order, inability to think clearly, blunting of memory, depression, irritability, drowsiness or inability to sleep. Incoordination of movements and slight changes of gait and speech, accompanied by dizziness, also persist. Once started, the disease progresses steadily without intermission. The initial disturbances increase in severity, new symptoms appear and increase in intensity often over a period of eight to twelve weeks, but occasionally as short as three to six weeks. At the height of the illness, a gross impairment of cerebral function leading to dementia may appear.

The Second Stage of the Disease starts with greater mental abnormality and unbalance, major clinical symptoms. There is general intellectual decline, followed by emotional weakness, very rapid in some patients, before a depressive phase becomes apparent. The symptoms and sequence of events vary considerably and can include an inability to recognise, loss of ability to carry out familiar, purposeful movements, and difficulties in expressing themselves in words. The patient becomes ultimately unable to continue with most of his daily routine activities. Characteristically, the syndrome may last from a few weeks to several months or, in some cases, may continue for as long as one and a half years. Reflexes alter, muscles become stiff or weak and movements are awkward. Shock-like contractions of particular muscles (myoclonic) in the upper half of the body are common, especially in this and the following stage.

The Third Stage of the Disease is marked by aggravation of the symptoms lasting from a few weeks to months. Most patients have a mere vegetative existence with gradual progression of the symptoms of the second stage. They are characterised by sound sleep, inability or refusal to speak, temporary paralysis and myoclonic and epileptic seizures. It is a kind of living death.

The Potential for Misdiagnosis

In the UK study, neuropathological examination is essential to the correct diagnosis of CJD particularly in the 5% of cases with stroke-like presentation and the 10% of cases with a duration of illness exceeding a year. It is possible that even strict adherence to the diagnostic criteria will miss some of these cases and there is justifiable concern that CJD may be missed in the elderly, especially where the "new strain" of CJD cases are involved.

To understand fully the current situation, it is important to know the classification and identification now used in the diagnosis of cases. For CJD patients, three diagnostic categories are in use:-

1) Definite CJD: histologically confirmed cases showing typical spongiosis.

2) Probable CJD: cases with a typical clinical picture and lasting under two years, but lacking histological confirmation. In this category are included relatives of definite CJD cases who, according to the clinical descriptions and testimony of collateral family members who knew them, also died of a similar disease.

3) Possible CJD cases: these were relatives of definite CJD cases but for whom clinical records, descriptions and testimony of collateral family members were lacking, while the information collected from other sources revealed that they had died of a dementing disease, similar to that of a verified case. Thus, where a demented patient was a relative of a definitely diagnosed CJD patient, in the first, second or third generation, that patient could be classified as a possible case of familial CJD.

Routine Diagnosis and Confirmation of CJD Cases

The problems of accurate diagnosis certainly add to the difficulties of conducting epidemiological surveys, making all the more important the use of all available diagnostic procedures, including electron microscopy of thin sections of brain, and the simple touch impression technique to confirm the diagnosis. A study should have been previously organised with the object of obtaining pathological specimens from all suspected CJD and other neurological disease cases for such confirmation.

The important clinical diagnostic symptoms of CJD are myoclonus and mental deterioration. Electroencephalograph

(EEG) is a technique for recording the electrical activity of the live brain through the intact skull. The technique is simple and gives valuable diagnostic information about epilepsy and encephalopathies, including CJD. It is considered sufficiently distinctive to help in the diagnosis of the disease. The underlying mechanism to explain periodic sharp wave complexes is unknown.

In about 50% of CJD cases, EEG specific pattern changes are important diagnostic indicators. In 25% of sporadic cases, however, periodic sharp wave complexes may appear only late in the clinical course, or, EEG activity may appear normal in as many as 25% of them. Where CJD has developed more slowly over a long period of time and some of its most characteristic elements such as myoclonus are absent, the EEG is found to stay within the normal limits. In almost all the BSE-strain CJD cases, the EEG pattern changes appear only in the advanced stage of the illness, when patients can no longer stand or walk. The observations that patients with CJD and prominent cerebellar symptoms are less likely to exhibit periodic sharp wave complexes may be secondary to reduced cerebral cortical involvement.

In the past, in a number of accumulated studies, a simplified schema for the clinical diagnosis of CJD was used as follows:

a. Definite cases: having mental deterioration, myoclonus and 1-2 cycles/second periodic EEG complexes with an illness duration of under 12 months.

b. Probable cases: having mental deterioration with myoclonus and 1-2 cycles/second periodic EEG complexes with an illness duration of under 18 months.

c. Possible cases: having mental deterioration with any type of movement disorder or EEG periodic activity with an illness duration under 24 months.

Laboratory Diagnosis of Creutzfeldt-Jakob Disease

It is commonly assumed that a post-mortem immediately provides the cause of death. That, unfortunately, is not the case with CJD. On visual examination, CJD brains usually appear normal, or, at most, show a mild to moderately diffused focal swelling of the brain and no lesions have been demonstrated in any organ outside the central nervous system.

Only a microscopical examination of the brain section can confirm CJD as the cause of death. Brain tissue is highly infectious and its examination therefore requires close adherence to an approved set of safety procedures. No short-cuts are permissible; corners cannot be cut. It is a time-consuming process. There is no alternative but to wait patiently for the necessary laboratory work to be completed and the final results become available. While, in most CJD cases, the pathological changes in the brain and spinal cord are obvious, they show up in a number of grades. The essential neuropathological pattern, however, consists of widespread degenerative processes with vacuoles seen in nerve cells in all layers. With the diversity of ways in which the disease presents, that should come as no surprise. Not all parts of the central nervous system may be equally affected. In earlier and less severe stages of the disease, the completely destroyed neurons may be few in number, although many of those remaining show pathological changes of an acute kind, consisting of shrinkage of the nuclear material, fragmentation and dissolution of the layer cells. In some cases the neuronal damage may be very widespread throughout the central nervous system, in others it may be localised.

Lesions have been seen in all parts of the brain, most commonly in the basal ganglia, thalamus and cerebellar cortex. In sporadic CJD cases, spongiform changes in the cerebellum are very rare. In BSE-strain CJD, on the other hand, there is extensive vacuolation in the cerebellum. This pathological finding is consistent with the leading clinical symptoms of the latter being problems with balance. This is the major difference and distinguishes sporadic cases from those of the new disease.

Significance of Vacuoles

The degenerative process is clearly initiated and caused by the infection. For many years, researchers have regarded the holes in the neurons as of major importance for diagnostic purposes, with everything else being unrecognised or ignored. The precise significance of vacuoles, their numbers and distribution is, as yet, troublesome and puzzling. In spite of the many advances in knowledge made in recent years, there is still much uncertainty as to what actually constitutes a hole in a nerve cell when viewed through a light microscope. The differences between normal and infected tissues can be minimal, making recognition and identification of the vacuoles extremely difficult. The spongiform change in natural scrapie, as well as being variable in its appearance, is never as extensive as it is in experimental scrapie.

The vacuoles result from the damage caused by the infection, the agent can incubate without their formation, and, therefore, the presence or absence of vacuoles is not a reliable indicator of SE. In the case of all the cattle in the UK clinically diagnosed as infected with BSE and slaughtered, over 20% (32,000 or more) were found to have no vacuoles in their brains and were, therefore, not officially included as BSE victims in the statistics. Whether this means that these animals were free from BSE (and had been clinically misdiagnosed) or that their histological examination had failed to detect the disease is uncertain.

The same reservations apply in human cases. CJD is not regarded as confirmed in the nearly 50% of clinically diagnosed cases where, although all the typical symptoms of CJD are present, no vacuoles are seen. They are, therefore, excluded from official records, leaving unanswered the question of how much reliance can be given to a clinical diagnosis in human cases based on the presence or absence of vacuoles. Were such diagnoses wrong, or were the histological examinations at fault for not going far enough to detect the the disease? To give credence to them and have these records show the true picture, these excluded cases must be further investigated.

It is now known that CJD and other related diseases are associated with the accumulation of deposits of PrP plaques in the brain. A reliable and accurate immunohistochemical technique for staining these plaques has been developed. In humans the presence of PrP plaques in suspected cases can be used to confirm the disease. It is proposed that examination of PrP plaques which are specific for CJD and other SEs should be carried out as an additional confirmatory test, in particular in suspect cases where there is a clinical history of SE but where spongiform changes in the brain cannot be demonstrated. It is essential that this test should be performed. Specificity of immunostaining of this antisera is very reliable.

Vacuoles in Narang's Disease

The cerebellum (the portion of the brain responsible for the maintenance of posture and balance) in BSE-strain CJD cases shows extensive vacuolation compared to that in classic CJD cases where there are very few if any vacuoles to be found in this part of the brain (Fig). Moreover, BSE-strain CJD cases all have PrP plaques in their brains. In all such cases duration is 12 months or more. Some correlation between the duration of the clinical course in these patients and the density of plaques seems to exist. Based on the clinical and histopathological differences, Len, aged 58, Elizabeth, aged 59, Helen, aged 62, and Brian, aged 47, all died of BSE-strain CJD.

Empirical as the age criterion may be, it was based on widespread observation and was accepted unquestioned, as a self-evident truth, by most medical scientists. CJD was a disease which could present only in the elderly - patients aged 50 and over. Persons under that age were, *ipso facto*, not suffering from CJD, similarity of symptoms notwithstanding. Uniquely in the scientific encyclopaedia, the virus was acknowledged to have recognised an "age barrier". That, at any rate was the accepted wisdom of the medical profession for many years and that credo, based on an unproven hypothesis, is not the first to have failed the test of time and the emergence of new data and factors. Unique as is this virus is in many respects, the power to select its victims on the basis of age is not within its capability!

Figures on Facing Page.

Fig.1 Spongiform changes in the cerebellum are seen as multiple small vacuoles in the molecular layer from few (a) to extensive vacuola tion (b). Haematoxylin and eosin stain, x 126.

Fig.2 Immunocytochemistry for PrP of a section of cerebellum from 59 year old case shows strong staining PrP positive plaques, x 80, and at higher magnification from 47 year old case shows several multicentric plaques with perivacuolar deposits, x 210.

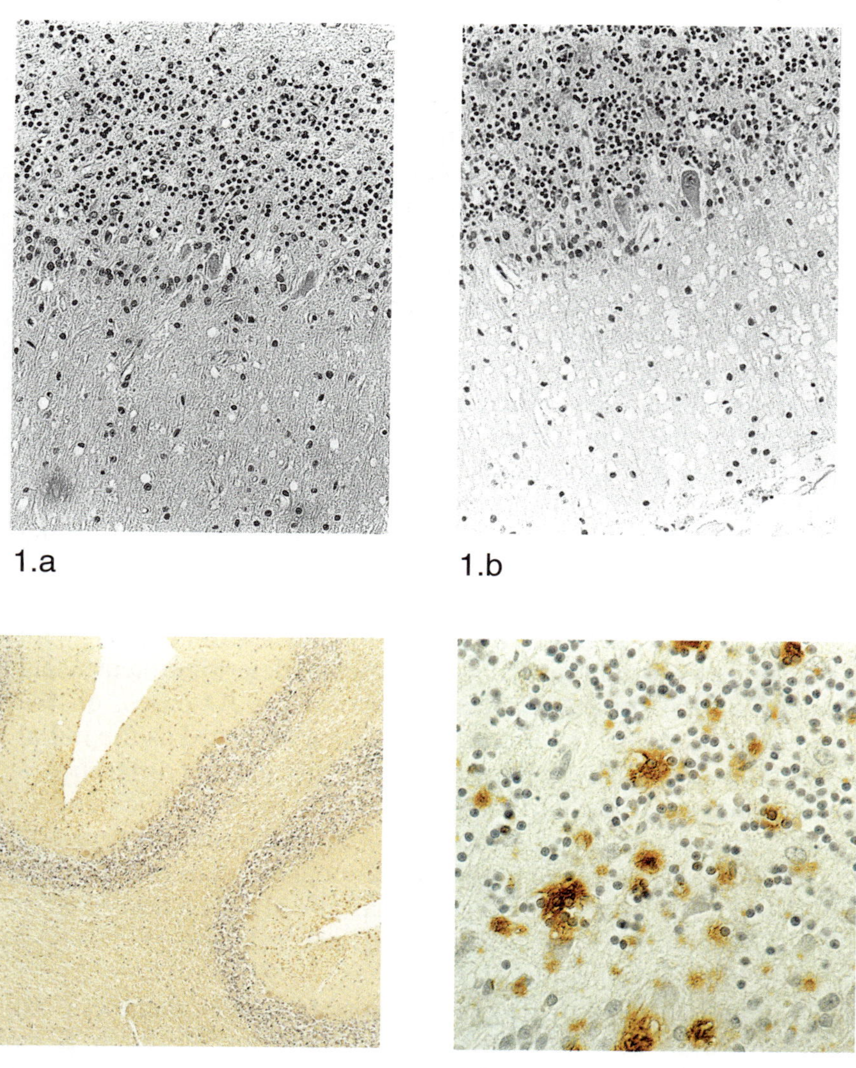
1.a
1.b
2.a
2.b

Classification of CJD Cases

All spongiform encephalopathies, regardless of their initial clinical symptoms and final pathological findings, are caused by the one transmissible infective agent (virus).

From world-wide epidemiological surveys, however, the existence of the following three main groups of victims has been identified:-

1- Sporadic: Sporadic cases form the majority of cases world-wide and, as the name would imply, no connection of any kind can be traced to link one with another.

2- Familial: Here two or more cases occur within the same family in one or more generations. These are estimated to represent between 5% and 15% of all CJD cases.

3- Iatrogenic: These cases form a small percentage of the incidence of the disease world-wide and result from accidental inoculation or the use of contaminated tissues in medicinal preparations and procedures as, for example, growth hormone prepared from human pituitary glands collected during autopsies, and in instrument and transplant cases. This is the only group for which there is, as yet, a scientifically-based explanation.

The clinical pattern in all iatrogenic cases begins with cerebellar syndrome - ataxia - with mental deterioration as a late manifestation. In the majority of sporadic CJD cases, on the other hand, mental deterioration has been observed as the initial symptom. Exactly why there should be this striking difference is not understood. The early age of infection in iatrogenic patients is not the only explanation: sporadic CJD patients with atypically early onset are identical to the overall population of the sporadic cases of CJD. The sporadic group has already been described in detail. The other two groups require further detail:

The Familial Form of CJD

A minority of all CJD cases occurs in family members. To account for such familial cases, some consider it to be a hereditary disease with a host gene termed PrP as its centre. This hypothesis originates from Nobel prizewinner Dr Stanley Prusiner, who suggested that the scrapie agent is composed exclusively of a protein, without a scrapie-specific nucleic acid. He termed this protein "Prion" (PrP). Surprisingly, the protein isolated was in fact found to be derived from a normal gene which did not differ in any of its biochemical or immunological features from the protein isolated from either normal or affected individuals. The same protein is found in all animal species. All proteins are composed of amino-acids: different proteins consisting of different combinations of different amino-acids and are coded by different DNA. The comparative structure of the PrP amino-acid sequence is almost identical in both humans and other mammalian species. This has been discussed in detail in my book "The Link".

Role of Mutations in the PrP Gene

Once it was recognised that PrP was a host-derived protein, molecular genetics entered the scene and a search began for mutations in the corresponding human gene among those families affected. In one sub-group of familial cases, termed GSSS, mutations were found in the PrP gene and this stimulated new interest in molecular genetics. It has been suggested that these point mutations observed in the PrP gene may cause the disease. In fact, different point mutations were found in different affected families, with more variations being discovered every year. The significance of these mutations diminishes as more and more varieties are found. Furthermore, our knowledge is limited: many other healthy families, or or those suffering from other neurological diseases, may have similar mutations. They have just never been examined. Sporadic CJD cases, which form the majority, do not have these mutations, thereby strongly indicating that these host-mutations are not part of the agent.

The enthusiasm over the last decade for regarding the mutation as the agent has waned. The discovery of yet more mutations will probably add little more to what we already know. They may well be predisposing: they are neither the agent nor an essential part of it. The same mutation has been seen in a number of first degree relatives of affected patients who are healthy into their 60s and even mid 70s. The important difference is that animals, inoculated with tissues from patients who have died from CJD, do develop the clinical disease, while animals inoculated with tissue from relatives without clinical disease remain healthy. There can only be one conclusion from this. CJD patients are carrying the agent, their relatives are infection-free. It is the agent which is the deciding factor.

Essential to the hereditary hypothesis is the assumption that a protein is the agent. There is no direct evidence to support this. CJD is infectious: hereditary diseases are not. Only indirect evidence has been used to support the mutation hypothesis. That mutation in the PrP gene is the cause can be easily tested in animal models. The sequence of the PrP gene has been well established in mice. There are several strains of mice with the same amino acid backbone in the PrP gene. Different strains of mice, however, when inoculated with the same strain of the agent, develop clinical disease with different incubation periods. Similarly, same strain mice inoculated with different strains of the agent have variable incubation periods, thus demonstrating that it is not the PrP gene that controls the incubation period. If the PrP gene does not control even the incubation period, how can it be said to initiate CJD by itself? This evidence suggests that there is another host gene or combination of genes which might control the incubation period.

I, personally, do not believe CJD to be hereditary but it may well, in some families, pass from one generation to the next as vertical transmission in the same way as we have experienced in AIDS cases.

There is no evidence that mothers are more frequently affected than fathers. Genealogical evidence shows skipped generations where there is no CJD case. All these have made understanding difficult. It may be that some families eat more brain tissues than others, since oral transmission of scrapie, kuru and CJD has been demonstrated and now there is the experience of the food-borne transmission of BSE to cows.

In animal exposures, where infection has been documented after oral feed, transmission was so irregular that the question arises as to whether the true portal was the gastrointestinal tract itself or through areas of mucosal abrasions. In some patients, the portal route of entry may be through bad teeth. Ulcerations in the lips, gums and intestines may also play a role since it is known that the disease develops with a significantly shorter incubation time where such ulcerations have been present.

There are only two reported cases of conjugal disease where a husband and wife both died of CJD within a few years of each other. If, as might have been thought, the infection transmitted in food, it would surely have been likely for many more such cases to have appeared.

Iatrogenic CJD

The risk of transmission of the infection by medical procedures brings with it grave implications. That it exists is clearly illustrated by the tragedy when some infected human pituitary glands were unknowingly included in the preparation of growth hormone, and its use in subsequent treatments passed on the disease. Cessation of the use of human glands in the preparation of such hormone will have eliminated this particular risk. The tragedy, nonetheless, highlights the problem and the virulence of the virus and the need for continual safeguards to prevent any similar occurrence. With no test yet being employed to detect the infectious agent in asymptomatic blood, tissue or organ donors, it is difficult to see how any such foolproof safeguards can be devised. It is an ever-present continuing risk and the implications are horrifying.

Nature of the Agent

The vital requirement is the identification of the true nature of the agent. Many transmission studies have revealed the existence of different strains of the agent and the agent behaving in the manner of a replicating infectious virus. The virus has some unique properties. There is no other virus with which it can be matched for comparative studies. Various assumptions have therefore been made based on indirect evidence. One-sided assumptions about the agent and the disease have been accepted as established facts, thus laying wrong clues, and misleading researchers.

Two structures have consistently been seen by the electron microscope (EM) in all SEs, both the experimental and natural diseases: 1) Scrapie-associated fibril (SAF) and 2) Nemavirus. Both are considered specific ultrastructural markers. While opinions differ as to whether the whole Nemavirus or merely its central core protein is the actual agent . This remains to be resolved and has been discussed in detail in my other book, "The Link".

Determination of the true nature of the agent is essential to the further understanding of the disease and the development of a diagnostic test and treatment.

*****

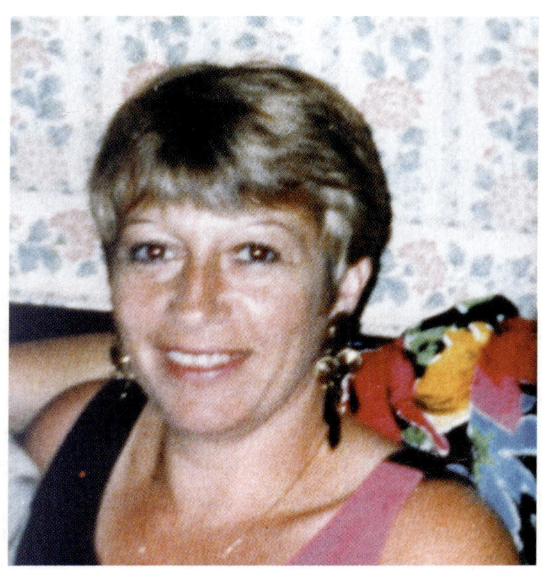

Anne Richardson

Anne Richardson, healthy, happy-go-lucky wife, aged 41, with one son, died from CJD in Liverpool in 1996. Ronnie, her husband who cared and looked after her during her illness, describes his experiences with medical staff and how his wife was snatched away from him by a dreadful disease. Anne started with depression, balancing and walking problems, typical of Narang Disease. To Ronnie's anger, medical staff seemed to blame him for causing her depression. After her death she was confirmed one of the first ten cases of the new strain of CJD. Anne was a blood donor.

I'm intelligent, even if I mightn't be well educated, but Anne was too sharp for me and that's why I loved her and that's why I married her. We were only married for ten years. We should have had another 15 or 20 years, but we didn't. A dreadful disease took her away from me. Anne was always happy and healthy. The only trouble she had was a few years ago, when she was treated for either a peptic or duodenal ulcer.

We've always been animal lovers. We'd often go to places like safari parks or the Zoo - that was our interest. We were out one day when she said: "Ronnie, I just don't feel right. I feel as though I've got a big cloud on my head and it's pushing me down". I said: "You need a tonic." So, I got her some tonic. I thought 'two days and she'll be sound again'. But, from then on, she didn't really want to go visiting and, on the odd occasions when we did bump into people, they noticed she wasn't her usual self and would ask: "What's the matter Anne?".

She didn't look right, she didn't sound right, she didn't walk in the same way she always had. I took her to see her doctor and he told her she was going through a nervous breakdown and prescribed anti-depressant tablets. That's what we were told and that's what we told her friends.

She had a tremor in her hands and her leg started to bounce up and down. That, we were told, could well be a side effect of the anti-depressants. I wasn't happy because they were telling me it was in her head and that it was the side effects of the tablets. So I thought 'okay, let's do away with the tablets and the side effects' and she stopped taking the tablets. Seven weeks after taking her off the tablets, she was worse than ever. At that time, Anne was at home with me.

Looking back, the hardest part is that we treated her as though she'd had a nervous breakdown and had to cure herself, so we were forever saying: "Pull yourself together for goodness sake". At one point I was on the verge of leaving her. I couldn't take any more, my head was bursting. I was just going to say: "Right, that's it". I couldn't leave her because I loved her too much. Then, after I found it was not her fault, it left me feeling very guilty. If only she had been here now, I would say to her: "I'm so sorry, Anne, for the way that we treated you."

So, I went back to the hospital, and I said: "Look, you're barking up the wrong tree. You told me it was side effects, it's not. I took her off the tablets for seven to eight weeks, and she is still as wobbly as ever. Her speech is worse and her confusion and ramblings are twice as bad. It's got to be neurological not psychiatric". I was told: "We've seen this before. We know what we are talking about, you don't".

I'm only a wagon driver, so I've got to listen to these people. But, in my heart and soul, I knew she was too strong for a nervous breakdown and it must have been something more. Well they wouldn't listen and they wouldn't do a brain scan. So after a couple more weeks I got so . . . . off, I said: "That's it, I've had enough now. Are you telling me I'm lying and I'm not telling the truth? Well I'll tell you, you're admitting her. Take her in. Don't give her any medication, no tablets, just watch her 24 hours a day and tell me what you see."

Ten weeks later she was admitted to hospital. By this time her walking got worse, her confusion got worse and they still weren't coming across with any answers. They did not treat her and gave her no medication but it was obvious to anyone that she was far from well, that there was something seriously wrong. All the time she was in hospital, I was getting more and more worried because the light and sparkle was going out of her. Although she always had a smile, it wasn't my Anne.

I said to the doctors: "Listen, you've got to do something. Here's what I want doing." They said: "No, you've got to do it our way." So I said if it's a problem of finances for your brain scans, because you're always whinging you're under-funded, she's in BUPA. Let's do it through BUPA. No more shilly shallying, let's get it done. Two days later, they still hadn't set the ball in motion.

On one occasion Anne was in the TV room in the hospital and, when she stood up she just fell and broke her nose, blackened her eyes, smashed her lip. I got a phone call to say: "Can you come in? Don't be alarmed, Anne has had a slight accident." So I went in to the hospital, and saw her in a terrible condition and said: "Will you do something now?"

Two days later, they did a brain scan and an EEG and on 1st December they got the results. When I went in, I was expecting them to say: "We know what it is, you were right. It is indeed neurological." I was expecting them to tell me it was a blood clot on the brain or a little pressure point or something, and when I went in to get the results, they said: "You were right, it is neurological." ***I thought 'thank God, at last they've found what it is'. I was so relieved I breathed a sigh of relief and asked: "What is it?" The doctor said: "Creutzfeldt-Jakob Disease."***

I didn't know what CJD was. So I said: "What medicine are you going to give her?" He said: "None, it's not like that. Do you know what Mad Cow Disease is? Well it's very similar to

that. It's called CJD. She'll just get progressively worse."

I couldn't believe it. He said they were going to transfer her to a psychiatric hospital and on the Friday she got moved to Walton Hospital. On Monday morning, I went in for a consultation with him and he explained to me what was involved. I said: "Okay, so I'm going to lose the girl. There's no treatment, no cure, but we must make sure her last months are as comfortable as possible." He said: "I agree with that." I said: "So I want an assurance from you that from now on I'm not going to be coming in here from work to find my wife all bashed up like has been happening in Broad Green on several occasions." He said: "Mr Richardson, we will look after her. She is in good hands."

That was at half-past nine in the morning and I was back at 6 that evening. There she was, in a wheelchair, with all her face bashed up again. She'd been in the bed with the cot sides up. She had wanted to go to the toilet and when she stood up, she just collapsed. As she tried to get hold of the side of the bed, she fell. She looked like she'd been beaten up. She looked like an ex-boxer and that was all due to the falls she was having regularly while she was suffering from this horrible disease.

Irene, her sister, told me what had happened and I said: "Go in the ward, collect all her stuff together. I'm discharging her." I went in and asked: "Who's in charge here?" and this chap came forward and said: "Me."

I said: "Well listen, that's my wife there. You told me this morning she was in good hands. I'm sorry but I don't think she is."

He said: "Mr Richardson, we're awfully sorry but these things do happen in hospitals."

"This happened all the time in Broad Green. Why has it got to be my wife? I'm not happy and I'm taking her home. Don't try and stop me, because she's coming home with me now."

He said: "Well we've still got more tests to conduct".

I said: "When you're ready to do tests, phone me and I'll bring her back". I just took her out of the hospital at half-past six in the evening, brought her home and she stayed at home till she died.

The doctor rang me two days later for a lumbar puncture test. I took her to the hospital and held her hand while they had her bent over on the bed and took the fluid. This test, they said, would help them diagnose that it might just be something else. After they did that test I carried her out and brought her home where we had brought the bed downstairs. ***I told the hospital people: "Right, that's it now. You're not touching her anymore, she's not your guinea pig. You've had all you're going to have, leave us alone now. I'll look after her myself."***

When we brought her home, her speech was slurred really badly. I brought Anne home from hospital on 4th December, our 10th wedding anniversary, and it was my 30th birthday on the 5th, so we had a gathering. A few of the family came round; we got a few bottles of champagne. Anne was sitting there and I gave her a glass of champagne with some orange and she sucked it through a straw. She was like a five-year-old child. You could see the excitement in her eyes. She was happy to be getting attention. But she didn't know why. She was elated at having her friends around and, although her speech was badly slurred, we could still understand her - although sometimes only with great difficulty and that made her frustrated and, at times, aggressive. She knew what she wanted to say and, when we couldn't understand her, she could get really aggressive.

See that doll hanging off the ceiling, the one with the ugly face? They are called expression dolls. That was Anne's doll, and she'd be lying in the bed, and she'd mimic it. Little childish actions, that's what she was reduced to.

Whenever Anne was asleep, we had a chair there and one of us was always sitting in it in case she tried to get out of bed. Still she'd get so far up and then just fall over. We had to keep an eye on her all the time. When it was time for bed, I used to get that couch and bring it round, take the cot sides off, and shove the couch round and I'd sleep on the couch so if she fell, she'd fall onto me. Once or twice, she was climbing over me in the night to go to the toilet. She was all floppy and didn't seem to have the strength in her body to do what she wanted. She was so independent it was unbelievable. I'd pick her up and I'd carry her to the toilet and I'd sit her on the toilet. She was sitting there for ages and she just wouldn't go.

About a week before she died, when she had been lying there asleep, she opened her eyes and she looked at me and she said:

"Ronnie, I'm frightened. I'm dying."

I said: "You've had a bad fever, and you've been delirious. You'll be all right, just go to sleep." I could see the reassurance in her face and she just went back to sleep. A couple of days later she went into a semi-coma. The night she died was horrible, it was horrible. Normally she was eight stone in weight but when she was ill she went down to about five stone.

Just before Christmas Day - and remember that she died on 5th January - she was sitting there, because we'd take her out of bed to try and ease her pressure points and move her around on the couch or whatever, and ***I said to her: "I love you, Anne" and she looked me in the eye and said: "I love you too, Ronnie."***

About a week after I took her home from hospital, Dr Martin Zeidler came from the CJD Surveillance Unit and asked all manner of questions. I answered his questions and he was here for six hours. I wanted to know just as much from him. I told him everything I could and did everything I could to help him. He asked my permission to take blood from her and told me: "What happens is you're born with this rogue gene. It could be genetic. This rogue gene splits and spins off or twists or whatever." So when he was telling me about this genetic thing he said: "You are born with it and you go through life and then it splits, spins off and creates problems. And that's how it comes about. In 99.9% of the cases, there are cases on either side of the victim's family with Alzheimer's Disease." I said: "Well I can put your mind at rest on that one because neither Anne's mother nor her father have ever lost anyone with Alzheimer's." He said: "Yes, but we won't know till we do the tests." He also told me that CJD only hits one in a million. My Anne was one in a million, wasn't she?

He had all these questionnaires. The number of questions was ridiculous. He wanted to know the ins and outs of everything and I answered to the best of my knowledge. I was 100% honest and truthful. I also gave my permission, as Anne's husband, for unlimited access to all her medical files from her GP, her psychiatrist, and from the neurosurgeon so that he could see the complete picture and history.

No hindrance was put in his way whatsoever because whatever he found out we wanted to know anyway. I did say: "If she dies of CJD I am going to make a hell of a lot of noise. He said: "I don't blame you." He obviously had to act within guidelines from his superiors. I don't blame him directly for me not getting the information I needed. I blame the Government for laying down guidelines for the CJD people in Edinburgh. ***As far as I'm concerned, they are saying: "Let us know, but don't tell them, they're only the victims' families". That's what makes me angry. Everybody else knew before me and I am angry about that.***

I told him: "If my wife is dying of this disease, I'll help you with everything I can and I'll assist you in your studies but, I'm telling you now, when my wife dies, if you want her brain, or any other little bits for your tests and your research, you can have them, but on the condition that, whatever your conclusions, I want every bit of paperwork you've got when you've finished, every last bit. Failing that, you're not getting her." He shook my hand and promised me he would give me every bit of information on my wife's case.

We had to cope with all this all on our own until only at the very end we did get some outside help. The last couple of days we got some nurses, but they just came in for half an hour. The problem was you were frightened to go to sleep knowing it was so close. About four days before she died, I was exhausted, mentally, totally, physically, emotionally drained.

Her twitches were getting worse all the time. She stopped going to the toilet completely. The doctor said her kidneys had failed, and he gave her something to start her kidneys. Because I felt she was in pain, she had morphine on the last two days. At the same time they tried to catheterise her but they couldn't get anything at all. After that, and when I saw the suffering that girl went through, I am going to make sure that these b.... pay for it, because they've hidden too much from us and they've been too deceitful. She should never have died.

For about four hours before she died, she was breathing very slowly. Her head lay at a funny angle and she had a weird posture lying in the bed. That's all she did. She just lay there. At the end, she wasn't really aware that you were around. We knew she needed something. If I had my way, I would have given her a big load of morphine and given her a kiss and wished her good night. I would not have dragged it out unnecessarily for those extra five days. It was not fair. She wasn't eating, she wasn't drinking, she wasn't going to the toilet. In fact, it's still killing me now, just talking about it. It's killing me and cutting me up inside and its making me more angry and fuelling the fire inside me because I want to kick some b.... I want to see some people made responsible for it.

I only got the full confirmation of everything on the morning of Mr Stephen Dorrell's announcement. Dr Zeidler did come back to see me after Mr Dorrell's announcement and that was when he told me, because up until then I still didn't know that Anne was one of these so-called ten.

When Dr Zeidler rang me, he said: "Your wife wasn't genetic." That was what had particularly worried us when we asked him if it was genetic, because Anne's son, who is 21, had a young baby of six months old. We were really worried that they might have the same disease. When he came out to see me a week or so later, I asked him: "By the way, is my wife one of those ten?" and he told me: "Yes, she is". That's how I found out. I had to ask him. He didn't volunteer the information.

None of them have wanted to give the information we've asked for. All along, we have been completely and utterly honest. We have given them free access to everything they wanted, and yet, at the end of the day, when we have asked for something back, they've pooh poohed the idea ... you're nobody, was their attitude. Even though I was telling him how frightened, upset and worried we all were, he showed us very little sympathy or human understanding. "It could be another six weeks before we get the results of these final tests. Don't you know how complex this whole issue is," he said. Even then, I only got the results after many frustrating phone calls and arguments. That, surely, shouldn't be the way.

When I first lost Anne I didn't know whether I was coming or going. I was so stressed out. I couldn't even go to bed.

I did ask Dr Zeidler: "What about BSE? Is there a connection?" He said: "I can't talk about BSE. I can only talk about CJD." He would not be drawn about BSE. He said: "I can't talk about it because, in all honesty, I do not know, but I will tell you anything you want to know about CJD."

Why should they put stumbling blocks in the way of the family when we were only trying to find out what'd happened to my wife? I needed the information I was asking for. I needed to know whether it was genetic so as to know whether or not to have Darren, my step-son tested. If they had said it was genetic I would have been on the phone to Harash straight-away and said: "Come down and test him. Test them all."

As far as I am concerned, she must have picked it up from something she'd eaten, something that's meant to have been fit for human consumption but wasn't.

So far as her teeth are concerned, she did have a couple of fillings and often had these recurring abscesses. That was because of her dentist. When he ripped the tooth out, he left a piece which he couldn't remove and that's where the abscess recurred and recurred. She had one missing tooth and one that was bad. It is on her records that she'd got an ulcer, I'm not sure whether duodenal or peptic, but in the 11 years we were together she showed no signs of it. In the summer before I met Anne, she had a really bad illness. It was to do with her stomach. It was a gastric thing that she had, but I can't remember the details.

Harash: Was she ever scratched by cats?

Yes, all the time. When I met Anne she had two cats and, during the course of our marriage, that grew to five and we had at least half a dozen stray cats from around the area that we used to feed in the garden. We built kennels for them. They very rarely ate a tin of cat food because Anne used to buy them stewing steak and cut it up. She often had scratches, raw wounds from them, the kind that break the skin, usually on her arms, but once or twice, when she would be lying on the couch watching the telly, and one of the cats might be on her chest, it would dig in and she'd get a scratch on the chest.

Harash: Let's talk about food now. Did she ever prepare soups and broths and things like that?

Yes, she would prepare ox-tail stew and dumplings. I know now that ox tails are part of the spinal cord and I can't understand why they are still selling them. We loved ox tail or neck-end stew and used to have that all the time. Hearts and pork chops with the piece of kidney attached was another of our favourites and, at least once a week, because it was my favourite meal, we had spaghetti bolognaise. At least twice a week, we used to get a Big Mac and chips and I would get a chicken burger and chips but sometimes I would get a Big Mac.

Anne used to love kebabs. Anne ate those until they were coming out of her ears. Nearly every night Anne used to have a kebab. I know I've never had a kebab in my life.

The reason I went public about Anne was that I wanted to find out the truth for sure and to have the truth made public and I don't care who's embarrassed because in a nutshell somebody has ..... up and they need taking to task. As far as I was concerned, I was led to believe she had a nervous breakdown. Then I thought to myself '... how many people are there in psychiatric units now allegedly suffering the effects of nervous breakdowns who are going to freak themselves out completely?'. Because people who have had a nervous breakdown may be led to believe that, in fact, they have CJD.

If the Government and whoever they are, the powers that be, were to lay the facts on the table and be honest then you wouldn't have all these people getting needlessly upset. Dr Zeidler did say to me, that, on his way to visit me, he had a nice piece of steak. That was ridiculous. Couldn't he have seen it? I told him I was going to make a noise and I didn't care who I upset. I had been upset by being robbed of a good woman.

Harash: Now tell me, did anybody ever try to sell you meat at the door?

Yes, and at work. I work in the building game, and there's always lads coming round with meat for sale, beautiful meat. I don't know whether it came straight from the abattoir or whether it came from a butchers or somewhere but it was knocked-off meat. I don't know anyone who hasn't bought it when its gone round. The man would say: "I have bought some nice big choice joints of meat and brisket. Psst. ... it's been knocked off, but it's from a proper abattoir."

Harash: Was Anne a blood donor?

Yes, she gave blood but she has never received blood herself. That was in Mount Pleasant in early 1980s where my sister worked in the blood transfusion centre.

If only I had known how ill she was, and how little time she had left. I certainly wouldn't have told her: "Get yourself together and stop acting stupid, otherwise I'm going to divorce you." I would never have said that. I wouldn't have divorced her. I was trying to shock her back to normality and it hurt me that Anne's family couldn't understand how it was hurting me and were blaming me for her having a nervous breakdown.

It even led to an almighty row and, after that, we didn't speak. They wouldn't visit me, I wouldn't visit them and if we saw each other in the street we turned around. Until then, we had all been a close-knit family but that changed and the hospital authorities didn't help and even added to the ill-will by their suggestions that some of Anne's troubles were my fault. They were trying to blame me for Ann's illness. That was at one case conference. I said: "Your case worker is meant to be looking after Anne and the feedback you're getting from her does not correspond with what I'm telling you. You are being told that when I drop Anne off at the day centre, she is wobbling and banging herself on the walls but, as soon as I am not there, she's all right. You're not listening to me. As far as I am concerned you are a psychiatrist and I have every respect for you and your profession but this woman, whom you have named, to look after my wife, is wrong. She's not worth a carrot and she's not fit to look after my wife. I want her off the case". So, he said to me: "What do you think it is, Mr Richardson?" I said: "Well, I think it's neurological". They all thought I was an idiot.

Naturally, the psychiatrist stuck up for his staff: "If you are going to speak to my staff like that I don't want anything to do with you."

I said: "Hang on, you're out of order. I want you to help me and help her, but you've put an incompetent person to look after my wife".

At the end of the case conference, he said to me that, out of all the interviews he'd had, he'd never been in a case conference in his life with so much raw aggression and it scared him. I said: "Well I'm sorry, but I'm not just an aggressive person. I'm an angry frustrated young man who's watching his wife go to hell in front of his eyes and he's not getting the answers he's asking for. On the contrary, he's being blamed for her illness. He said: "Well, as far as I am concerned, judging by what we have seen today, from your attitude, and from what we have been told when we've spoken to Anne's family and from the feedback from Anne herself, I think that Anne's problems lie at home." I said: "Okay you're saying her problems lie at home. There's only me and Anne at home, so what are you saying?" He just looked at me and said: "Precisely".

It's too late for him to apologise now but I hope he has learned his lesson. I never asked him for an apology. When Anne was being cremated they sent two nurses from the psychiatric unit to the crematorium. One of them gave me a handwritten letter from the psychiatrist apologising to me. I reckoned that was enough. I haven't spoken another word since to that man. Well, let's hope the next time he gets someone in like that, he'll know what it is and be a bit more understanding.

Yes, well you can understand my frustration on being told that all her problems were in her head and had been caused by me. The reason I said that I thought it neurological is that knowing Anne as closely as I did, I knew she was too strong to have a nervous breakdown. She would deal with whatever arose and she was so efficient and strong-willed she could run rings around me. I knew she would never allow problems to accumulate or overwhelm her. If there was a problem, she faced it: she never ran from it.

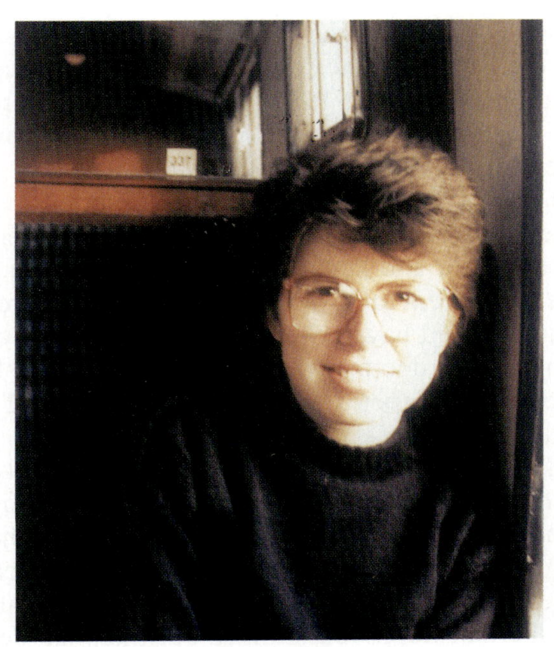

Alison Margaret Williams

Alison died on 17th February, 1996, aged 30. The cause of her death, established by post-mortem, was bronchial pneumonia brought on by "new variant" CJD. The first signs of a developing illness, although their significance was not realised at the time, were first noticed by her family in 1987. These initial signs included so complete a change in her personality and attitude, so noticeable and worrying to her mother, that Alison was quickly referred to a hospital for tests for diabetes and thyroid deficiencies. These, however, proved negative.

Until the start of her illness, Alison, from Wales,was an "outdoor girl ". She loved skiing, walking and sailing. Being of a happy and cheerful nature, she had many friends. She was a perfectionist in all she did. She loved her family. Her health had always been good and she had no significant dental history. She had been a regular blood donor. Here, Alison's father talks to Harash and tells how the developing disease gradually took over Alison's life and brought about her death and has left an irremovable scar on both his life and the life of Alison's brother.

Alison started at teacher training college in Wrexham in 1985 studying for a BA honours degree in Business Studies. That was a four year course which she started two years before my wife's heart operation in August 1987. Alison, however, packed up College in the July but, at the time we put this down to her anxiety over her mother's health.

From the end of September 1987 Alison started to go down. She became very restless and both my wife and I were worried about her behaviour and lack of interest and reluctance to meet people. She often went up to her bedroom and sat there for hours by herself and would have nothing to do with either of us. My wife took her to the doctor who arranged for tests to be carried out in hospital for diabetes and thyroid problems. These tests proved negative.

From 1987 onwards, she held various temporary jobs, but had to be driven there in the morning and picked up at night. She appeared to have completely lost her confidence and her interest in life. In July 1992, she was treated for a suspected nervous breakdown. The GP gave her some anti-depressants and by December she had improved slightly but then she deteriorated even further. She lost pride in her appearance, general hygiene and dress sense and just wanted to wander round in a jogging suit.

Before she became ill Alison was a perfectionist as far as her appearance and clothes were concerned. Throughout 1993, even though she did some hill walking, her confidence deteriorated even further. From November onwards she was counselled by her doctor to prepare her for the loss of her mother.

In April, 1994, when her mother died, she coped well with the situation and in the August obtained a job as a clerical assistant and worked for the period of a month. One day she collapsed at work. She believed that everyone was against her and in September, 1994, she went into hospital for a fortnight where she was treated for acute depression by the consultant psychiatrist.

When she came out of hospital she seemed to have improved but, as the year drew to a close, she completely lost interest in her appearance and personal hygiene such as washing and bathing. At that time my son, David, was working in South Wales. Alison and I used to go down on alternate weekends to see him. She showed no interest in going round the shops when we went with her to Liverpool, Chester or Manchester, which she previously used enjoy. On each occasion she sat or lay in the car.

She became very choosy about food and would go into a restaurant, order a large meal and only eat a small amount of it. She would eat the vegetables, but would not eat the meat.

From October, 1994, Alison became unsteady on her feet and her walking was a sort of a marching gait, kicking her feet out in front of her, something like a goose step. In November she went out with a friend of hers on the hills and walked about 150 feet up the mountain and completely froze. From then onward she lost all interest in everything.

From November, 1994, Alison complained about pains in her calf muscles and in her ankles, wrists and finger joints. She also complained about feeling cold all the time and insisted on having the central heating on 24 hours per day, winter and summer. That resulted in room temperatures of 20 - 25°C. At the end of the year, she was not washing properly and would run bath water and then not use it. Her memory started to deteriorate and she became forgetful. She developed a habit of going to bed and not pulling the continental quilt over her but used to get inside the cover. On two occasions when I went to Caernarfon to post a letter, she vanished out of the house for two to three hours and that caused me a lot of concern and anguish.

From 1993 to February 1995 Alison attended a number of Government Training Schemes to help her return to work. On the last occasion she was placed in one of the sheltered workshops in the area to carry out clerical duties. Prior to her decline she was computer literate. She worked for one day at the workshop and for the rest of the week just sat in the office looking out of the window. She did not do a thing, so the manager of the workshop sent her back to the ITEC Centre at the end of the week. The manager at the Centre sent for Alison and me. She was in tears at the meeting and was asked to explain her attitude. She did not give any reason at all but just said that she could not cope and complained that she was cold. The manager gave her two months off and asked us to come back. When she got home after the meeting, she screamed her head off at me and said: "I am very, very ill." It was obvious that she had lost her confidence. She knew that there was something wrong with her but could not explain what her problem was.

By March, 1995, even if it was just a simple letter, she could not cope with the computer and ended up thumping the keyboard and losing her temper. She also used to rub her forehead a lot but could not explain what was wrong with her. From January, 1995 onward she was losing weight and by April of that year she had lost approximately two stone and was admitted into hospital in May, 1995 with suspected anorexia.

After a week's treatment, the Consultant Psychiatrist informed me that it was not a psychiatric problem but an organic one. Alison's case was referred to a Consultant Neurologist who transferred her to the Neurological Centre in Liverpool in June, 1995 for further tests. The Consultant thought that it was the rare disease, Huntington's Chorea. David and I were counselled for the Huntington's Disease genetic tests and we were told that it runs in families. The implications of the genetic tests, which could affect David, were fully explained to us and we both agreed to this genetic testing.

Prior to going into hospital in May, Alison gave all her clothes away and I can only assume that she had given them to a charity. Before she went into hospital she did say that clothes were evil. That was a strange comment when you remember how she previously enjoyed having so many beautiful clothes in the wardrobe.

From June to November 1995, her walking and memory deteriorated. She seemed to be in a world of her own and on several occasions she became hysterical and screamed her head off and would stamp her feet for no reason at all. That could go on for 10 - 15 minutes at a time - no doubt it appeared the fear of the unknown. This happened on one occasion when travelling by train from Chester to Bangor going through tunnels when a train was passing in the opposite direction. She could not cope with any noise whatsoever - the dogs barking, television, freezer, washing machine and would scream at the dogs and switch off the freezer, washing machine and television.

From the time she came out of hospital, she needed support for walking by holding my arm and ultimately became wheelchair bound. Because of her confused state in the morning, when she got up out of bed she would sit on the edge of the bed and wet it and she needed assistance to get dressed and undressed and had to be toiletted. I brought a bed downstairs so that she could lie on it in the afternoons. In no way could she keep still. She used to toss and turn, her legs and arms flailing out all over the place and would grunt and groan all the time and there would be excessive head movements. We did not know if she was frightened of something or suffering from hallucinations.

In August, 1995, the Genetics Nurse at the hospital met David and I and explained that there was a grey area regarding the genetic tests that had been carried out on Alison and that we should meet the Senior Registrar in Medical Genetics from Cardiff. ***He confirmed there was definitely a possibility that Alison had CJD which could not be confirmed until her death. If this was the case, it was probably not Huntington's Disease. The matter was then discussed with our GP who sympathised with our tragedy if it was CJD and he gave Alison a life expectancy of 3 to 12 months.***

Alison gradually became worse. She was incontinent and would cry frequently. She developed sudden jerky movements, she could not keep still, her speech was slightly slurred and she would also go stiff and tense. She suffered from loss of memory and would only get half dressed.

In September, 1995 she went into hospital for about three weeks to give me a rest. By the end of October, I found that she was unable to walk, and I had to give her assistance when she went upstairs by walking behind her, and walking in front of her when she came downstairs, lifting her foot off the step and placing it on the next one. On some occasions, she would scream her head off. By this time she was having problems with loss of memory. I told the doctor that I could cope no longer and she went into hospital into the Young Persons Disabled unit in November, 1995. From then on, her condition got worse and she had to be fed. She screamed at the nurses, spat at them and attempted to bite them. She could not keep still in bed. She was thrashing about with her legs and arms, tossing and turning, and even with bed rails fitted she was able to throw herself out of bed, and she was confined to a wheelchair permanently. The sister told me that when they took her to the bathroom one night, Alison saw herself in the mirror and screamed her head off. From then on they always covered up the mirror.

When the Consultant Neurologist examined Alison in November, 1995 he was adamant that it was not CJD, but a rare case of Huntington's Chorea disease. Our local MP was interested in the case and the Consultant briefed him. Once it had been established at the inquest that she had the new variant CJD, he phoned the MP with an apology

You could not hold a conversation with her. You had to do all the talking, the only sign of recognition would be a smile when I visited the hospital every day and fed her. Her condition deteriorated further and she spent her time in a wheelchair or bed.

The sister told me that ultimately Alison would lose the use of her muscles in her tongue. I contacted my GP about that seeking advice and wanting to know if she would be in any pain. He said: "No." I told him that in no way did I want her to be put on a drip and I was told that she would die within a matter of 7 days and would not be in any pain. Confirmation letters were sent to the doctor and sister stating that Alison was not to be put on a drip and my signature was witnessed.

Our GP told me that Alison's body would have to go the CJD Surveillance Unit in Edinburgh and that her brain would be removed. I wrote to him confirming that David and I were agreeable to this, and that, if required, any of her other organs could be removed and used for medical research.

I also told the sister that once the muscles in the tongue went 1 would no longer feed Alison as I thought that there was a special way of doing it and if I fed her and she choked I would never be able to forgive myself.

Two to three weeks before Alison died she went blind, and would just stare into space, her face just like a mask. There were no reactions from her but she still continued to thrash about with her legs and flick her legs up and get the back of her knees on the rail and lift her bottom up and slide onto the floor. The back of her legs were bruised even though cushions and pillows were placed around the bed rails.

During Alison's stay in hospital the sister in charge of the unit admitted to me that she had never treated a patient with suspected CJD before and she said it was just a case of loving care.

On the Sunday before Alison died, she went into a coma and could not use the muscles in her tongue. They could not feed her and the sister told me on the Monday that she was near the end of her life and I spent nearly all of my time in the hospital. Her breathing pattern changed over the last week of her life, and, during the last few hours, it was as if she was gasping for breath. During that time her hands, arms and cheeks turned blue and she died on Saturday at 12.15 am on the 17th February, 1996. The doctor certified that she was dead and her body was removed by the undertaker for transportation to Edinburgh.

Whenever I visited Alison, I used to hold her hand and talk to her and you would see a smile on her face. From the time she went blind until her death, I used to do the same thing but there was no movement of her eyes and there was no pleasure shown - not even every evening when I left the hospital and gave her kiss on her forehead.

David and I are grateful to our GP for all the help given to us over the years, and also the consultant doctors who were involved with Alison's case. The care and attention in each hospital was excellent and the way in which the nursing staff cared for her to the end of her days helped David and I through a most difficult period of our lives.

The theory expressed by the doctors was that when Alison was in College, she went into one of these fast food cafes as a student and ate infected meat there, sometime during 1985 to 1987, when there was all that problem with meat.

We were not a great meat-eating family. We used to eat a lot of fish, chicken, pork, lamb and only occasionally, beef. We used to have steak and kidney pies and food like that occasionally at home when we went sailing at weekends and on motorways when we visited Little Chefs or the like. The meals would commonly be a cheese burger or beef burger.

At no time did Alison have any blood transfusions or treatment with any growth hormones. She was a regular blood donor and gave blood at least 4 - 5 times after leaving school. Her teeth were excellent. She did have a number of fillings over the years. When she was in hospital, however, her gums started bleeding because a very hard toothbrush was being used.

The initial shock and anguish of Alison's condition was unbelievable, made all the worse by the uncertainty as to its cause. ***Once established that there was a possibility that it was CJD, the outlook was grim and every time we visited the hospital we did our best to make Alison happy. Then came the dreadful day when she died. That, in one way, was a relief because we knew that she would not suffer any longer. We then had to come to terms with our grief, me losing a daughter aged 30 years old and David, his sister. This is the time when relatives need the most help.***

With David being away from home Monday to Friday, I spent many hours by myself and virtually became a recluse. On some days I did not want to meet anybody. Apart from collecting the newspapers from town and shopping for food, I used to sit at home with the dogs all day doing nothing. I had many sleepless nights and horrific dreams about Alison. I developed a bad chest infection for a period of six weeks having been so rundown. From July onwards, I started to pull out of the fit of depression and David and I became more active. It was then I decided to do everything in my power to help other people who found themselves in a similar situation to the one I had been in.

At the time of Alison's death doubt was expressed that she had CJD. ***In March 1996, the Coroner's Officer informed me that she had died of a rare neurological disease. That caused yet more anguish and uncertainty. Having consulted my GP, we were told that David would have to submit himself for further genetic tests and, not recognising the implications, I did not know which way to turn. I read an article in a paper referring to a seminar being organised by Dr Harash Narang in Newcastle on the possible links between BSE and CJD.***

I contacted him and we discussed Alison's case history. He stated that, in his opinion, she was a victim of CJD caused by BSE. That helped to relieve my worries about it being a genetic disease. I attended the seminar and it left me in no doubt that there was a link between BSE and CJD.

A couple of weeks later I received the post-mortem results stating that Alison had died of bronchial pneumonia brought on by the new variant CJD. David and I have lived through a devastating experience and it will be years, if at all, before we will be able to come to terms with Alison's death.

We have received information and help from the CJD Surveillance Unit in Edinburgh and have collected a lot of information via the Internet. That has made me determined to spend the rest of my life as a care person with the CJD support network to help people who find themselves in a similar situation.

Looking back on my own experience, I can only pray that some means can be found to lessen the strain that uncertainty brings. The not knowing just what it was for so long, made it all the worse and, even after her death, they were still unsure. Yes, it was indeed CJD. No, it was not Huntington's. That, for David's sake at any rate, was a blessing.

Each Health Authority should ensure that their consultants, doctors, nurses and ancillary staff know how to deal with CJD victims and their relatives and not give them the impression that they are stumbling in the dark.

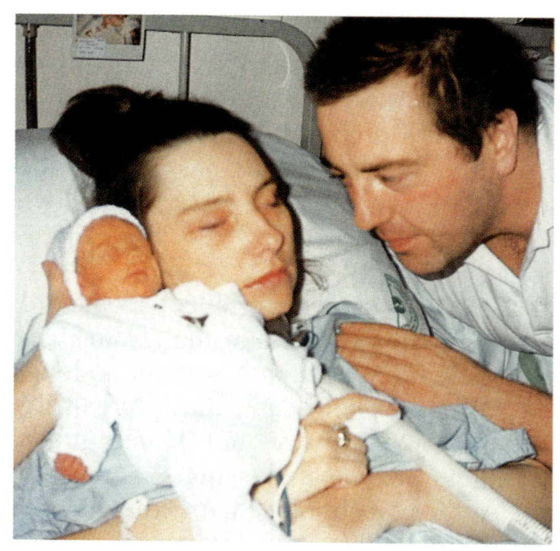

Michelle Bowen

Michelle Bowen died aged 29 from CJD on November 25th, 1995. Three weeks earlier, her baby, Anthony, was born by Caesarian section while Michelle was in a coma. She lived in Manchester with her husband, also called Anthony, 36. They were married for nine years and already had two daughters, Natalie, five, and Jacqueline, nine. Anthony describes to Harash losing his wife to CJD - and his fears for little Anthony. He also tells of the enormous problems he had in getting diagnosis confirmed and the hidden agenda behind the BSE/CJD crisis.

Michelle was born in her grandfather's pet shop. Michelle and I were married in 1986. We had first met twelve year previously when she was 17. We used to speak to each other on the CB radio. She had a very strong personality. We were fairly happy and then, suddenly, about 18 months before Michelle died, I saw changes in her behaviour. She started showing signs of going off the rails. Back in 1993, I remember looking at her and sometimes thinking that she appeared to be mad. There was just a mad stare in her eyes.

Her writing became shaky. She used to forget who I was. If we saw a lorry while we were out driving, she would say: "I wonder if that's Anthony." I would say: "Well who am I?"

She suddenly decided in 1993 that she had had enough and didn't want to live with me any more. She just took the kids and left. I was devastated. I just couldn't believe it when she left. I would see her two or three times a week and I kept in contact for the sake of the kids. But she was letting everything go in her home: she was not paying any bills. She wasn't really coping on her own. She wasn't eating at all - except ice cream. She wasn't sending the kids to school. She said she still loved me, but she couldn't live with me.

We had had our ups and downs and I didn't think we would get back together, but we did. In August 1994 she came back. She always seemed to be rushing about a lot. She would say: "Let's go here, and let's go there, let's move away." I would ask: "how can we do that? I haven't got the money". She said: "Let's do the house up" and in November and December 1994, we put in a kitchen. As soon as that was finished, she wanted to start doing something else. She seemed to be manic depressive, never happy with what was there.

Just after Christmas, she stripped all the hallway and decorated the bedroom on her own. She did a good job. Then she said: "Come on, let's have a look at fitted units for the bedroom". I was earning fairly decent money as a truck and crane driver but there was not a lot to spare. I said I didn't have enough money in the bank and that was it. She never ever asked again, she seemed to have forgotten all about it and never mentioned it again. She didn't seem to mind. That shocked me: from wanting to spend everything and after my having said: "No," she just stopped and lost interest. That marked the start of her illness, though I did not realise at the time that she was seriously ill.

She stopped going out. She started forgetting things. She was suffering from a mild depression. Her mother was ill, suffering from vascular dementia. Michelle had been going to the hospital three or four times a week, talking to a neurologist, psychologist and brain surgeon about her mother's condition. They weren't going to let her mother out, but instead were going to transfer her to a care home because they said there was no-one at home to care for her. In about April 1995, her favourite uncle died of cancer and that added to Michelle's depression all this time. We assumed her depression was due to her mother's condition, the stress from coming back after the break-up of her marriage, and her uncle dying of cancer.

Although she wasn't a pet lover, in April she turned up with a puppy, a pit bull terrier that was only going to create trouble when it got bigger. I didn't want a dog, and I was a bit unsure of his temperament. I knew Michelle couldn't look after it and could not understand why she had got it.

One day that Spring, Michelle went upstairs with loads of tablets, and said: "I'm going to do myself in." She was adamant she was going to take them. I said: "You take them, and when the kids come in, what am I going to tell them?" She said: "You can look after them better than me." I talked to her a bit more and she calmed down. At that time she wanted to take her own life.

She was always having emotional outbursts of anger or crying. I asked her what was she depressed about. "Is it me, the house or the kids?" I asked. "I don't know. It's not you, it's not the house, it's not the kids," she said. She knew something was wrong with her, but she didn't know what. I thought she was worried about the house and suggested to her: "We'll get an extension built; no hassle. We will be all right." But that idea didn't seem to help.

We found out that she'd missed her period at the end of May but she said: "I can't be pregnant". Well, I said it could be stress - she was a bit depressed and again I asked her what she was depressed about. "Is it me, the house or the kids?" In the summer, she was told that she was pregnant but she denied it and refused to believe it. Then she started having more emotional outbursts of anger or crying.

In June, for her 29th birthday, I arranged we would go out for a meal. She didn't even bother getting ready. If I said something, she just let me do what I wanted. She had lost interest in everything. She was getting bigger, and at the same time she was unsteady on her feet. One of her aunties accused me of not giving her enough money to get clothing. I explained that I gave her money. I had got her a new pair of shoes and she only had them a day before the dog chewed them up. The dog was messing everywhere, and I was coming home from work and having to clean it all up.

On top of that, she stopped cooking tea and I had to do that as well. About August, her auntie said Michelle was not well at all. We took her to the doctor's. He said that she was suffering from depression, either because of her mum's illness or because of the pregnancy. Then, we noticed she was becoming very unsteady on her feet. Her auntie said: "You'll have to get her a decent pair of shoes." She had loads of shoes, she just would not wear them. She just couldn't walk without someone holding on to her. It was as if she was drunk. She was walking from side to side, and had also developed a jerk in one of her shoulders. To get to the kitchen, she would grab onto the chair and settee. On one occasion, Michelle came out of the house and was walking towards the car and she ran past it into the gates. She just couldn't stop herself, just took off on the little slope and smashed into the gate.

In September, she started leaving house doors open - even the front door. She forgot how to start the car. She was not cooking, cleaning or anything. I had to give up work. Jacqueline was eight and Natalie was four at the time. I thought Michelle was suffering from a mental illness. She didn't have any strength left, only when she was angry. She used to physically grab the kids over nothing. She started hallucinating. She stopped going to bed and started sleeping on the couch.

One day, I had taken the children to school and she suddenly started shouting: "Where are the children?" Her eyes were glaring. You would think she was on some kind of drug. I had first wondered about that the year before. She used to have sudden rages when her eyes were popping out of her head.

She had an appointment with a psychiatrist who told her she was suffering from a very bad depression. We were alternating between seeing the doctor and the psychiatrist. Michelle always used to pull herself together for these meetings. She had a fear of being put away.

She became very slow at eating. But I made her eat because of the baby. I got a phone call telling me to bring her down to see a neurologist in October. At that time, I had looked after her on my own for six weeks. She was driving me crazy: I couldn't keep up with her. She denied living here with me in the house. She didn't even remember she had put in the new kitchen. She was either asleep or just bursting out and jumping up.

I didn't have a clue what was up with her. The day she went to see the neurologist, she peeled skin of her feet like a banana. I told her to have a bath before she went to see him. She wasn't brushing her teeth, she hadn't been washing herself since August. She was also buying clothes which wouldn't fit her. I took her to the neurologist on October 13th. They did a brain scan and found nothing. They suggested that it was something mental. A week later, they suggested that it could be something physical, such as a tumour. She had to stay in the hospital.

We didn't take anything with us. She just shrugged her shoulders and said: "Don't leave me here." But they put her in a ward with other patients. That came as a shock to me. Within two or three days, she was in a room on her own because she had struck a patient and hit a couple of doctors and nurses.

Michelle's auntie had read about the CJD cases in a newspaper. We put it to the doctor. He said that it could not be ruled out and said: "That was a possibility." The paediatrician examined her and said she did not see any danger for the baby and was quite happy to leave the baby for the time being. Michelle was on a long list of drugs - everything. She was still speaking, but not very coherently. They did an EEG and it was irregular. They didn't tell us it was CJD. She seemed to be perking up a little bit. But now I realise that, while she wasn't getting any worse, she wasn't getting any better. She just stayed the same. After being able to walk her into the hospital, I found that she couldn't walk at all. She was not eating and that all happened within three weeks. With all the drugs they were giving her, I said it was no wonder she couldn't walk. I wanted to take her out and let her have a smoke. They said: "No." I couldn't take her out in the wheelchair.

The medical staff, for reasons known to themselves, wanted a list of family members who were and weren't to be allowed to come into her room. I got quite stroppy with them. I said that they had to let anyone come in who wanted to see her.

Not long after going in the hospital, she actually bit through her lip. It was swollen. Someone should have just put her out of her misery. I would have done that. She was going from one thing to another. They said there was no pain with this disease, but I think she was in pain all the time.

We would be talking, and we told her to lift her hand up if she could understand us. She did that once, and then she never did it again. They said they didn't know whether she could understand or not. It was just her body shutting down. I took the children to see her three times. She did remember the children. She was very low, you couldn't understand her. She was trying, but words were not coming.

Three weeks before she died, she started having fits. They phoned and told me they were going to have to take the baby. The drugs they wanted to give her would harm the baby, they said. They had been giving her steroids and she was bloated. They had hoped they would take the swelling out of the brain. I asked: "Are they working?" The doctor said that they had not kicked in yet. They were doing EEG every couple of days. They had moved her three times, the last time right next to the office so they could watch her.They did a Caesarian section on November 2nd. The baby was due to be born on January 18th. On the day of the birth, they didn't ask me if I would like to go in.

Dr Martin Zeidler turned up from the CJD unit, and asked me to come back the following Monday and bring as many people who knew Michelle. He asked us a load of questions for two hours. I asked him what he thought the trouble was. He said: "Yes, I think it's CJD." He advised us and said not to go to the press for all the trouble we would get into. "You will get harassed," and he said: "people will get hold of the information about your wife and make a major issue of it. But that's up to you."

He spoke to my sister and, straight-away, she said to me, "Get straight on to the papers - they are covering something up." She asked him: "Did she catch it breathing the air?" My wife was dying. I was going to end up on the dole with three kids, one who might not live because he was born so early, so to just say: "Don't go to the press," was asking too much.

They took blood while she was ill and said they wouldn't know for certain whether she had CJD until they did a post-mortem test. They wanted to know whether any of her family had ended up in a mental institution. For the last nine months, she had been like a dithering lunatic. I asked him:

"Would she get any better before she died?" He said burial arrangements meant I couldn't view her. I said she was Roman Catholic and wanted to be buried. He said a specially designed coffin would be required if we were to view her. They have to be put in - I think he said - steel boxes.

We didn't really know about beef. We were still eating beef. Dr Zeidler said: "I still eat beef," and, "There's no connection with beef. CJD had been around for centuries. They don't know how you get it. No. There's no connection with beef".

She was in a coma for three or four days. She woke up and tried to speak, but she sounded terrible. She had a big white tube sticking out of her throat. She was starting to get stiff. Her hands had gone straight. She never showed what I believed, after reading the book given to me by Dr Zeidler, were CJD symptoms. What was the point of giving me that book?

Then I thought she could have caught it from the beef, and I started worrying about the kids and myself. I don't care about the beef industry collapsing. Why do they want to save it? They never save anything else, they never saved the shipbuilding industry. But the Tories are farmers, aren't they? At the time, I just thought of Michelle. She had been unlucky.

They said they wanted to bring the baby down to see his mum. I showed her our baby. Michelle couldn't speak, but I told her: "We've had a little lad", and she smiled. Michelle recovered from the Caesarian, and was all right for a few days but then needed surgery. That was it. She never recovered after that. She stopped speaking. She kept getting infections, and I was asked whether they could stop treating her because they were just prolonging the agony, although they would still feed her. I said: "If that's what you think is for the best, stop treating her." Five days later she died, on November 25th. They phoned me to say that they were very sorry, she had passed away.

They said they would have a post-mortem done. On the Monday, I demanded to see her, and I went into the Chapel of Rest. I was stroking her hair and kissed her on the forehead. A man who had let me into the Chapel of Rest went berserk. He forced me into the toilet to make sure I washed my hands. I felt absolutely terrible. I wasn't really worried until he said: "It is very contagious when they die."

Why didn't someone tell me that I was not supposed to touch her body. I thought: "Oh God, I've put myself at even more risk." I was frightened to death. I went away and then went into the toilet and started throwing water into my mouth to clean it. I organised the funeral. The blokes were frightened to pick her up. They picked her up the morning that she got buried. She had not been eating, and they seemed to be struggling with the coffin, so what was in there I don't know. I don't know whether Michelle was in the coffin or not. They had told me I wouldn't be able to see her in her coffin. I wasn't allowed to see her, was I?

Harash: I don't believe the agent can jump to people, otherwise many more people would have been infected within families. At one time, pathologists didn't think it necessary to take the precautions they now do, even when carrying out a post-mortem. Frankly, I think a lot of these people who were with you at the time from the hospital and the undertakers were mistaken in much of what they told you, but, of course, they wouldn't have had much experience of this situation.

I had not seen her since the autopsy. They assured me that they were only going to take little scrapes of skin and little scrapes of the brain. They said you wouldn't be able to see. I wasn't in the position to be able to see, was I? Then I found out they had taken the placenta away, which I had never been told. ***They then called me down and told me my wife had died of CJD. I said: "What about the kids. I've got a nine year old, a five year old and a three-month-old baby. What's the chances of them or me having CJD?" He said: "With the two older ones, virtually impossible, but with Anthony, there was a 50-50 chance."*** He said I could have a test done, but a lot of people didn't like to know these things. He then went on about other diseases and said that people's lives were spoiled when they had found out they were ill

Sometimes it's nice to know if you've got the disease and sometimes it's not. But if they tested me and I had the agent in my body, I would just worry when the symptoms were going to start. Sometimes, I am a bit worried myself. I was telling my sister recently that I thought I was hallucinating. Maybe that is only my imagination working and not an early symptom.

Harash: Many patients do have hallucinations.

Sometimes I think they are just waiting for me, Anthony or one of the girls, to just start going down with the clinical s ymptoms. They should be testing people, I suppose, but they would go berserk to be told the worst. Wouldn't they? If you tell somebody who is criminally-minded that they have only got so long to live, and they're going to die a dirty, horrible death, he's just going to take the law into his own hands isn't he? It would be anarchy, wouldn't it?

In 1979, I worked in an abattoir where I was working with the offal. They slaughtered the cows upstairs, and I was working in a place called the 'By-products'. We wore protective head-gear so that our hair was not going in the food. We were given gloves, but you couldn't handle the stuff with the gloves on, so, we didn't use them. We were actually working with the intestines and the sheep's bellies. I was dealing mostly with the cows. Some of them were pregnant and carrying foetuses. They were heavier because they were pregnant, and more money was paid for them. Sometimes they had an almost full-grown calf in them. They used to sling the calf and the foetus aside and these were used for dog food. Michelle used to work at a butchers when she was about 18 or 19. She worked there before and after we were married in October, 1986. There she was handling raw meat,things like mince. She would clean it and cut it using a slicer. She has also worked in a cake shop, as a debt collector, behind the bar in the bingo, selling lingerie, and on a market stall selling flowers.

We often ate sausages and burgers. While they were out - her and her cousin - they used to always be having cheap burgers. She did used to take the kids to burgers shops. She probably consumed a lot of burgers when she was working on the market stalls - about 1989 and 1990 when she had trouble with her teeth. She could have had dodgy burgers at the time she was having trouble with her teeth. In the late eighties, she had had a lot of trouble with her teeth. She had one filling which broke and left her with a hole in her tooth, but she was frightened to go to the dentist. Maybe that's how the infection entered her body. She used to buy mince and burgers, used to get them made thick from the local butchers and freeze them. She used to do spaghetti bolognese and such like with it. Often she would buy on a Saturday from the indoor market. Very rarely we ate liver. She used to eat kidneys.

I would like to know how all this came about some day. Michelle was counted as one of ten new strain of CJD cases. The day after the announcement in the House of Commons in March 1996, Martin Zeidler phoned me at 8.30 pm. ***He asked whether we wanted to come up to see them, or whether they could come and see us. I started to swear. I said: "Why didn't you come and speak to us two months ago.*** You must have known Michelle was one of the ten." He said: "Well, yes." And then he started to say that there are a lot of people who think their relatives are in the ten but they are not.

I asked: "Who are the ten?"

He said: "That's patient confidentiality." I said that if they wanted to, they were perfectly free to give out my name.

"Oh we can't do that," he said.

I asked whether they were ringing all the ten families.

"Oh no, no, no," He said.

So I said: "You do not want us to get together, do you? You don't want us to know each other, do you? You want to keep us divided." I said: "I'll see you in court and I put the phone down on him." I have been to see a solicitor, who's looking at pursuing a 'duty of care' line. But I am just trying to get on with my life, and trying to put it behind me. I don't feel angry, but I can't forgive them for what they have done - giving us misleading, wrong information.

I know my story is probably one of the worst because of the three kids, but there is more than me who need to be heard. Ask yourselves, we do live in a free country and yet, we aren't allowed to know what's going on?

I had spoken to you (Harash) before you sent me the Mail on Sunday Night and Day article of 17 December 1995. I read it for over an hour one night. You are quoted there as saying that it was definitely a BSE infection - by the way she was acting, her symptoms were certainly those I'd seen in BSE cattle. Our Government admitted it after four months.

I do know you have got a test, and I can't understand why, if there is a test, they won't use it? Why don't they test all the cows, why just cull them?

Harash: How do you feel now about the whole thing? Are you going to forgive them when you know your wife died of BSE?

No I am not going to forget or forgive them. I am just trying to get on with my life and trying to put it all behind me. I don't feel angry but I can't forgive them for what they did when they misled us.

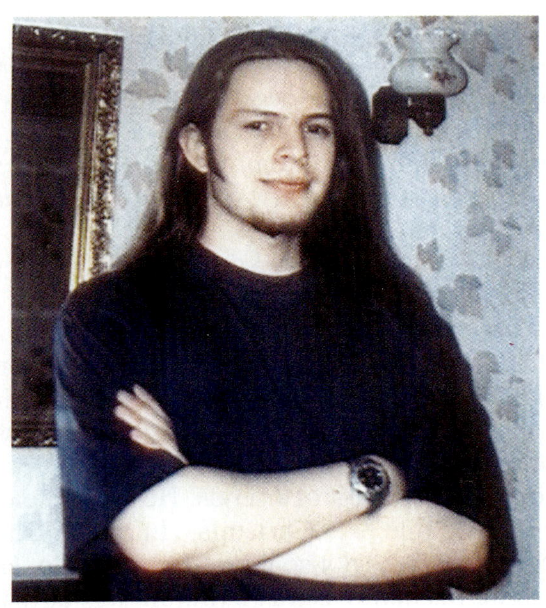

Peter Hall

Peter Hall showed the first symptoms of CJD at the age of 18. He died, aged 20, in February 1996. Six months later, a coroner said it was "more likely than not" that his death had been caused by eating contaminated beef before 1990. Peter, of Chester-le-Street, County Durham, was a vegetarian from the age of 16 but his favourite food as a youngster had been beefburgers. Dr Robert Perry, consultant neuropathologist of Newcastle General Hospital, told the inquest: "Most neurologists would link CJD to the BSE epidemic, but would probably not say so in public."

Home-shot video shown on television of Peter struck down as a teenager by the crippling disease provided an early powerful image of the devastation that CJD wreaks.

After repeatedly being told by doctors that Peter was too young to be suffering CJD, his parents asked Harash to perform a urine test. In January 1996, I confirmed that Peter had CJD before he died. This confirmation prompted a full post-mortem.

The acknowledgment that Peter died of the "new strain" of CJD, sparked a new urgency in official investigations into the link. If I had not tested Peter, the authorities might not have admitted the existence of the new atypical strain of CJD. With Peter's case, the Government began to accept for the first time BSE as the likely source of the infection. In doing so, they were merely confirming the validity of what I had been publicly claiming for several years, in the face of continuing and regular official opposition and discouragement.

Peter's mother, Frances, explains how a happy, healthy teenager was brought down by the disease.

Peter started at Sunderland University in September 1994 and enjoyed being there and spent spare time playing in a heavy metal rock group. He was reading environmental studies. He was obviously coping and passed the exams in December. He went out a lot, and had a lot of friends. He was a healthy young man and he seemed fine over Christmas. In January, he appeared a little off-colour. He was not so interested in his appearance and stopped washing his hair. He was living in digs at that time and he told us that the plumbing was not very good. He was coming home every weekend, and I said that so long as he gave it a good wash when he was home, it would last out the week. Then, I noticed he was not washing it much at home either, unless he was reminded. This was really unusual for Peter, because he was meticulous about his appearance. He liked scruffy jeans, but was always immaculately clean. His hair was long, well past his shoulders, and he was very proud of it.

At about the same time, I noticed his appetite was not good. He seemed to be losing a bit of weight, but I put that down to living away from home. He also seemed quiet, although he was carrying on pretty much the same as usual apart from that, but he seemed to be coming home more often. It reached the stage where he came home on Thursday evening and did not go back until Monday afternoon. He did not seem to want to go back.

One Monday morning, I left to go to work but had forgotten something and came back and heard him crying upstairs. I went up and asked him what the problem was. He said he did not like university, did not like the course, and did not want to go on with it. I had a good talk to him and thought I had it sorted out. I told him it was best if he could finish the course because there were not really any jobs going. He calmed down a bit.

But alarm bells were ringing. While visiting the doctor's about something else, I mentioned to her that I was a bit worried about Peter. I described what he was like, that his appetite was poor, that he seemed very down. She said that it sounded like classic depression, perhaps caused by the pressure of going to university, and meeting new people. She said to send him over for a chat next time he was home, but I could not imagine him suffering from depression. He was not the depressive type. He always took life as it came. He was a quiet lad: he never had highs and lows. He was always very even-tempered. His friends would say that Peter was the one who calmed down situations, that he never lost his temper, never fell out with anybody. He was just very even-natured. From being a little boy, he was always jolly. I found it difficult to accept at the start that he was depressed.

I always jump to the worst possible conclusions; it is part of my nature and immediately feared it was something worse. I had in mind CJD. I have had a horror of it for so many years. That was one of the first things I thought it might be. I knew about BSE from having seen television programmes on it. I had a horrible premonition, not of Peter, not that it was going to affect my family directly, but that something really horrible was going to happen. It just seemed obvious to me that this new disease, if it had jumped from sheep to cows and then to zoo animals, if it could jump these species barriers, it could jump to humans.

I first heard of it in about 1989. From then, I banned all beef from the house: sausages, burgers, everything went out. Peter became vegetarian in 1992. He may have eaten beef from 1989, I don't know. I just stipulated that if any of the family ate beef, they did not eat it in the house because I was not going to be responsible for buying it. I just did not trust it. They used to call me 'the mad cow' at work, because I used to say to people, "Please be very, very careful with beef. It's got this new disease and I just have a horrible feeling something bad is going to happen with it." All my friends will tell you. I was really so worried about it at the time that it is ironic that Peter is the one who actually got it.

My husband, Derek, loved beef but, from then, I would not buy beef. That caused moans and groans at first. When I used to buy burgers, I always bought good quality, the kind that said on the packet, '100 per cent beef'. When a product said: '100 per cent beef', I presumed it was minced beef - not bits and pieces. The same applied, in my mind, to sausages and mince.

I suggested to my doctor that it could be CJD but she said it was very unlikely. She calmed me down a bit but, in March, he packed in university. Just before Easter, he was due to go to the Isle of Arran on a field trip, and it all came to a head. He had left it until the last minute to pay for the trip. He was due to go on the Saturday and went on Friday to pay his money. I thought he was all right and, if he was depressed, going away on a field trip with people his own age could do nothing but good. I actually took him and put him on the bus. He rang me about 2 o'clock. I could hear he was in a pub. He just said: "Mum, I haven't paid my money." I said: "Well, why?" He said: "It's not worth it." The phone went dead, and I did not know where he was. He came home about 9 o'clock and, by then, I had imagined the worst. That was it. He just did not go back to university any more. I rang them to say he was ill and they deferred his course and said he could go back the following year.

After a while, he was staying in bed most of the day, while I was at work. I would give him his breakfast before I went out and leave him a meal. He would just lie about most of the time. I dropped one of my days at work and so had four days at home with him. He was put on anti-depressants.Then I noticed that his hands were trembling. It was that kind of movement he could not control. The hand tremor was quite pronounced. The only other thing.... you know if you put your foot in a certain position how your leg starts to go like this (she demonstrates her own foot bouncing up and down with foot half-raised off floor) but if you said to Peter, "For goodness sake, put your foot flat on the floor", he would only stop for a short time. I rang the doctor from work one day. I was so worried. She said that it could be a side-effect of the anti-depressants. He had been quite sleepy before he went on to them but as soon as he started on them he did not close his eyes for four days and four nights. I was up all the time too. The doctor altered the medication and, within a week, he was suffering unbearable pain. We went back again and the doctor put him on to Prozac which seemed okay. There did not seem to be any improvement but there were no obvious side-effects. He just slept, although not normally because he was up so much through the night, going to the toilet a lot.

The symptoms were building up and I became more and more worried. His appetite was very poor and his taste was changing. He had never been one for sweet food, but he started eating a lot of cakes and sweet things. He had liked fruit and vegetables but now seemed to be wanting whatever was easy to eat. He was not talking much. That was quite alarming. He never said he was ill. He was still walking, but more slowly. All his movements were slower. His short term memory was absolutely atrocious but I could not convince the doctor how bad it was. She said it could be a symptom of depression. It was just unbelievable. If he was watching the television, he could not remember what he had seen minutes before. He would be watching it, his eyes moving with the screen, but he could remember nothing about it. It was the same with a meal. If you asked him what he had just eaten, he just would not know. If I gave him a list of things I wanted from the shop, by the time I had reached the fourth one, he had forgotten what the first one was. And Peter, from when he first talked, had had an excellent memory. He had an excellent memory, so this change was particularly alarming.

By late April and the beginning of May, he wasn't walking as quickly as he had done but otherwise, apart from his tremor in his hand, he was okay. The only conclusion our doctor could draw was that he was in a deep depression. Then, at the beginning of May, three weeks after he started on the Prozac, he had a raging temperature. I had never seen anything like it. He was sitting in the chair, absolutely soaked from head to foot. His hair was wringing, his clothes were soaking wet, and he just looked awful. But Derek had just had flu and so had my elder son John, so I assumed that Peter had just caught flu and just put him up to bed. The next couple of days, he just lay around. I was still at work then, so I just left him in bed. I left him his dinner and said: "Stay in bed until I come home. I'll be in early." He stayed in bed for about three days.

I stopped work on a Thursday. That day, I went up and got him up and when he was coming down the stairs, he could not walk properly. His balance was totally gone. He took a lot of time to come down the stairs.

That was the last day he went out. His friends rang to ask if he wanted to go swimming. He said he did, so I asked them to keep an eye on him, because he was a bit shaky and not very well. Off they went. When they came back, I asked if he had been all right. They said: "No." He had changed, gone into the swimming pool but just stood at the side. He had not moved, just stood there and held on to the side. When he came back, I asked him whether everything was all right and he said it was.

There were times when he used to cry, but it is difficult to tell whether he was aware of anything. Peter was the type that would never like to worry me. I do not know whether he knew and did not want to tell me, or whether he was not aware. On the Friday, he was no better and I decided to stop the Prozac. By Saturday morning he looked worse. The woman next door is a physiotherapist and I asked her to have a look at Peter. I said: "Just look at the way he is walking, there's something desperately wrong." He looked as though he was trying to walk thinking the floor was inches higher than it was. It was like the rolling motion when people are on boats and cannot get their balance. She said: "If I was you, I would ring the doctor."

It was a weekend and the doctors hate coming out but I thought I could not worry about it all weekend. I had to ring. An emergency doctor asked what medication he was on. When I said Prozac, he said Peter had all the classic side-effects of Prozac. He told me to stop the tablets and see my own doctor on Monday and have her change the medication. I cannot say that did much to restore my confidence. Anyway, the day passed.

On Sunday morning, when I went to wake him, I looked at him and, unbelievably, his mouth had changed shape. He had always had perfect front teeth, very even, but when I looked at him they had crossed and his mouth seemed to have become smaller. I panicked then. I said to Derek that I was going to have to ring the doctor again. I know it is more than they say it is. Fortunately, when I rang, it was a doctor from our practice, and he came out. He tested Peter's reflexes and co-ordination. He did not say anything about his reflexes, they seemed to be okay, but his co-ordination was totally gone. At this time, Peter was still walking. He looked as if he was drunk. The doctor said it was more than depression. "I think you need to see a neurologist straight-away." He rang me on Monday and said there was an appointment for Peter on Tuesday.

We went for his first appointment in May. A neurologist examined his reflexes and co-ordination again. He asked Peter questions. He was still able to answer on his own, but slowly. The neurologist said he would make an appointment for a CT scan. He suggested I contacted our GP about making an appointment with a psychiatrist so as to try to work from both perspectives at the same time. Peter had a CT scan the next Friday. They said it was normal, nothing untoward at all. I suppose in a way it was a relief. I thought: "Well, it's not a brain tumour." He had an appointment with the psychiatrist the following Wednesday. He sat Peter in a chair and asked questions, which Peter did not answer, so I had to answer for him. Peter actually sat and went to sleep. The psychiatrist said: "I don't think its a psychiatric problem, but we'll get him in for assessment."

I took him the next day to the psychiatric hospital. He had been there three weeks when his memory was so shot that he could not find his way from his bedroom to the toilet, the door directly opposite. He could not remember the number of his bedroom. If he came out of the toilet and you did not watch for him, he did not know where he was. The same lady used to give him his meals every day, but he could not remember her from one day, or even one hour, to the next. He knew us, but he could not remember anybody new. He was having problems with his legs, and he could not walk very well.

They wanted me to leave him there. There was no way I could leave him. He was like a baby. He did not know anybody. He was like a stranger in a strange land. He became upset when I was not there. He was totally frightened all the time. I stayed with him. I went there early in the morning and I stayed with him until he went to sleep at night. We just left him when he was in bed and I went back the next day. They just more or less watched him, but it was totally the wrong atmosphere: people were there with breakdowns. It was totally the wrong place.

He was sent for an EEG. From his symptoms, I thought the EEG would be really erratic, but we were told there was no abnormalities at all. Because the tests were coming back normal, it was even more worrying. What was it that they could not detect? I was suspecting CJD more by then. They tried giving him high doses of thiamine, because there is a depressive illness which can be caused by a lack of thiamine. He had thiamine injections and thiamine tablets, which did nothing whatsoever, apart from causing Peter to develop a dread of needles. After three weeks, the head psychiatrist sent for me and said he had spoken to Peter's neurologist and they had decided it definitely was not a psychiatric condition. It was definitely neurological. He needed to go to another hospital for further tests.

I asked: "Is there any possibility it could be CJD?" He looked at me as if I had two heads, and said: "No, of course not. He's the wrong age. The time span's all wrong: with CJD it's six month from beginning to end. He would be a lot further along the road by now."

They ran a full battery of tests over a week. Starting with an MRI scan which again was normal, they did bone marrow tests, a chest X-ray, an endoscopy, and took samples from his bowels, spinal fluid and blood tests. Every time anyone came in the room wearing a white coat, you could see Peter cowering because he knew they had needles and he was terrified.

That was the worst part, having to sit with him when they were doing these tests. I had to sit and look into Peter's eyes, keeping hold of his hands and say it was going to be all right, knowing he was in pain. He was trusting me, and I was letting them do these things to him. He became like a child, and, like a child, he trusted me. At the end of the week, they said it would take six weeks before all the results came back. Three or four different neurologists came over to have a look at Peter, but they had no suggestions to make. I was told to take him home.

By now, Peter was having hallucinations. He hated open doors. If you left the door open, he used to sit and look very frightened until you closed it. When he was in the chair, he used to pretend he had a gun. He used to say: "There's snipers in there." He was so frightened. Sometimes, it took me an hour to calm him down. I had to sit and cuddle him. He was having horrendous temperature fluctuations, cold one minute and red hot the next. One day, he was freezing cold down one side and red hot down the other. It sounds ridiculous, but it happened. He had a quilt over him and he pulled it up one side. I said: "Peter, what's the matter?" He said: "I'm cold." I said: "Well pull the blanket up over you." He said: "No, I'm only cold at this side." When I felt him, one hand was red hot and the other was freezing cold. The doctor said it was part of the condition. I thought, 'Well, what condition? We haven't established what he's got yet.' His head had started lolling by this time. He could not sit up in the chair properly. His condition deteriorated a lot in the six weeks he was at home. I would sleep in the doorway of his bedroom, because he seemed to need to go to the toilet a lot, and I was frightened he would fall. The doctor suggested putting Peter onto a drug for epilepsy to calm him down and help him sleep through the night. He started off on a very small dose and that helped him to sleep a bit.

During these six weeks, they brought me a wheelchair but I determined not to use it. I was going to keep Peter on his feet. No way was he going to be in a wheelchair if I could help it. He used to get about by putting his hands on my shoulders, and I would hold him around the waist. I would walk backwards, and he used to follow me. I was still managing at that time to get him into the bath - with great difficulty. I used to have to dress and undress him by this time but he grew steadily worse until by the end of July he was in the wheelchair permanently.

At the end of six weeks, I rang the neurologist. He said the results of the tests were all negative. "Everything's normal. Nothing showing up at all." I said: "Where does this leave us?" He asked for Peter to be brought back to hospital for some tests to be re-done and in the last week of July, they did more tests. ***They had a seminar when I took him into a room where there were about 40 people. They were, presumably, doctors,*** but I do not know whether there were psychiatrists or whether they were all neurologists. Peter was in the wheelchair and his symptoms were described and demonstrated. I later asked if anyone had come up with anything and ***I was told: "No. No-one had anything to offer". Derek asked again whether it could be CJD and we were told that it was not.*** The neurologist asked if he could bring a paediatric neurologist to have a look at him. He said he knew Peter was slightly older than a paediatric specialist would normally see, but this man was very knowledgeable. I said: “Bring the Pope if you like, I’ll let anybody see him.” He came and examined him again and they ran a full range of blood tests again. He was also tested for Huntington’s Chorea which was a horrendous thought. I had three weeks of hell with that. They won’t do the test without you seeing a geneticist. I wouldn’t let them tell Derek. I was living on a knife-edge again. Logically, I knew it wasn’t, but, by this time I was in such a state.

Apart from you, Harash, and my own family members, I seemed to get no comfort or reassurance from anyone. There was nobody offering any help at all. We were just told they didn’t know what it was. Our neurologist said: “The only thing I’ve seen vaguely like it was a girl we had in here a few months ago. She died”. I asked if they ever found out what it was. He said: “No.” I asked if I could get in touch with her parents, thinking that maybe talking to them would help. They had been through the same thing: their daughter had died of a mysterious disease. I was later told they had been in touch with them but they did not want to speak to us. I just had to take their word for it. I do not know whether they actually contacted them, but had I been in the same position I would have wanted to talk to somebody. After Peter died, I really wanted to talk to somebody.

By this time, the beginning of August, we could not manage Peter at all. The day we had taken him back into hospital we had to carry him down the stairs, and he was a big lad - six foot tall. The doctor said they would have to find him somewhere to go. I said: “He’s not going into a nursing home with old people. Suppose I take him home and carry him up and down stairs on my back. He’s not going in there.” The doctor said that home was obviously not the right place, as we could not give him any treatment. He suggested the respite ward of Earl’s House hospital, where I would be able to stay with him. I could nurse him myself there and that was what I wanted. He had picked up a bug. He was very sick for two or three days, and losing weight fast. I thought we were going to lose him then, but he threw that off and started eating again.

He was having great difficulty controlling his head. I was finding it more difficult to feed him. He was having problems swallowing. I had to start feeding him while he was laying down. I took him out in the wheelchair as much as possible. Somehow, I managed to keep him clean and tidy. Derek used to come, and we coped. But Peter was definitely losing weight. In September, he was desperately ill and I thought he was dying. ***The doctor asked about a post-mortem. I asked whether we would learn something from it. He said not really, and I could see no point if it wasn't going to help find out why Peter was dying, so I said to leave it.***

There was more and more about CJD on television and in the newspapers and the more I heard about it, the more I thought there was no way that was not the same thing as Peter had. I asked the doctor again in December. He said: "I don't think it is, but I can't hand on heart say it's not."

After he went away, I thought, "That isn't good enough." ***I said we were going to have to contact Dr Narang who had been mentioned in a newspaper article, to see if he could do his test. As it happened, Derek had heard Mr Ken Bell on a radio programme and knew he was financing Dr Narang's test. So he rang Mr Bell and was put in touch with Dr Narang.*** I contacted Dr Narang, and I told the ward's staff nurse what we intended doing and asked her to tell the doctor. She said he did not know about the test, but had no objection in principle. Dr Narang came out that day and arranged to have the samples done.

People kept asking whether we were sure it was not CJD and could only would answer: "I thought it was, but I keep asking and asking and they say it definitely isn't. What can I do other than ask? I can't say: 'I'm not a doctor, but I know it's CJD.'"

Peter also developed a chest infection in December, and I rushed him to hospital. They said I had to be careful how I was feeding him. I had to make sure he was swallowing properly. He was okay for about a week, but then he had another chest infection. I got him pulled round again, but they decided that the chest infections were caused by food going down on to his lungs, so I could not feed him. Over Christmas, I could not give him anything to eat at all. It was dreadful. He was having water and saline drip. He was just ticking over.

Early in the New Year, we had the result of the test from Dr Narang. It was CJD. Dr Narang at this stage advised us that another EEG should be done. In cases like Peter, particularly where the symptoms start differently, the EEG pattern does not show abnormality until a certain stage of the disease has been reached and even then it's just what, medically, they term "a slowing down" pattern that is observed. So Dr Narang told us what to expect. Dr Narang also told us the importance of a post mortem and how much there was to be learned from the results.

I told the doctor of Dr. Narang's conclusions, but he would not accept them. He had a meeting with Dr Narang and afterwards said that we have to keep an open mind. ***I told the neurologist that Dr Narang had suggested another EEG and also that a post-mortem must be done. They took Peter over for another EEG, but they again said there was no abnormality. There was a slowing down, which was what Dr Narang had expected.*** So the result of the EEG test did not come as a surprise to us. Our neurologist agreed that a post-mortem was to be done.

Peter had been on drips for three or four weeks by then. He was so thin, it was horrible. I asked what were they going to do. They put a plug into his stomach to feed him directly. I knew it was not doing him any good, but I felt slightly happier knowing he was not hungry. He had had nothing to eat for all these weeks: it was horrendous. But at least he was receiving some kind of nourishment. He had started jerking a bit, his feet were moving. It was not all the time, but it was definitely an involuntary movement. He fell off a chair. We were told that Peter could not feel, and could not hear us. But when you spoke to him and stroked his arm, he smiled. I am sure he was aware. It worried me when people spoke about his illness in front of him. It is horrible to talk about someone dying when they are in the same room. He could definitely hear. His eyes used to go to the door when someone was coming. He followed you with his eyes. He was not blind and he was not deaf.

The Saturday before he died he was laughing at a joke. Derek was with us, and he went off to sleep. After about 10 minutes, when Peter had gone to sleep as well, I woke him. Later, Derek took Peter's hand and said: "Isn't that bloody typical, ten minutes I'd been asleep and your mother comes and wakes me up." Peter started laughing hilariously. He definitely understood what was said.

He could not talk at all by now. He used to raise his eyebrows, and that was how we communicated. That was a signal that he knew what I was talking about. I asked if he was suffering any pain. They said he was not, but to make sure they would give him diamorphine. That affected his breathing, and he used to go very blue. This started the day before he died. I had not been home for ten weeks. It was a lovely, frosty February morning, and Derek said: "Come on, let's go and have a walk." We told them not to disturb him and let him have a couple of hours sleep. When we went back after 20 minutes, I saw that he had gone blue. They gave him oxygen and within half an hour his colour was back to normal.

I had thought again about having a post-mortem. I had agreed to have one by then because we knew it was CJD, but it had to be confirmed and Dr Narang had told it was a must. They were not going to accept the CJD result from the urine test without it being confirmed by a post-mortem. I knew Dr Narang was due to go away abroad within the following few days, and I wondered whether to make them wait until he came back. I was becoming a bit neurotic about it all by this time. Derek phoned Dr Narang and told him what was going through our minds. It was a surprise when Derek heard Dr Narang's words: "I will postpone my trip. Keep in touch."

Peter was obviously deteriorating. By lunchtime, you could see he was going. He went very blue. His breathing just slowed, as if he had forgotten to breathe. They had asked us previously whether, if he stopped breathing, we wanted them to go into the 'crash routine', which could break his ribs. He would then have to be rushed down to the other hospital. We said: "No, there's no point. Just let him go peacefully."

About two o'clock, he just faded, peacefully, just the way he had lived. Didn't cause any bother. And that was it. There was just one last flutter, just as if a butterfly had passed under his ribs.

We then had all the fuss with the procedure afterwards. The ward GP came down, and we signed the forms for the post-mortem. They laid Peter out. We went back into the room. The vicar had come, and then Dr Narang. We waited until the undertaker came. He came and took Peter away to another hospital. He told us later he was concerned: he had not known what he had been handling. He had been told simply that there was a body to take for post-mortem, so he treated it the same as any other death. I rang Dr Narang to tell him that I thought the post-mortem was to be on Friday. I told them strongly that Dr Narang had to be there. They were a long time bringing his body back to Chester-le-Street. The coffin was sealed, which I had said I wanted. I was told: "You've got no choice. They will seal it at the hospital and then no one will be allowed to touch it again."

The neurologist wrote on the death certificate, 'pneumonia', followed by 'degenerative neurological condition?'. When we went to the registrar for the death certificate, she said: "I can't give you one." This was because of the question mark. I said there had been a post-mortem and we had arranged the funeral, for two days later. The coroner said there was no way the death certificate could be filled in. I asked: "What happens about the funeral? Everything's arranged. People are on the way, flowers are arranged. What's the procedure now?" I was told that the burial could take place once the inquest had been opened. She said: "If it comes to the push, in a case like this, have the funeral without the burial. Have the burial later on." That would have meant going through it all twice. She said that it would probably not come to that. We had to go to the coroner's office on the morning before the funeral and give a full statement covering Peter's illness from start to end, everything that had happened at the hospital, and what had been put on the death certificate. Derek had to go that afternoon to the inquest's opening at the coroner's court. I was unable to go. The funeral was to be the following day, and we had not finalised it. They opened the inquest, and the doctor had his knuckles rapped for the way he had filled in the certificate, and for letting the body be removed without the paperwork. It emerged at the hearing that the undertaker had had a right carry-on. He had gone to the hospital where they conducted the post-mortem to pick up Peter's body and asked them to sign the release form for the burial. No-one there would sign it, so he brought Peter back to Chester-le-Street and had gone to our GP who would not sign it. She had not seen him for months. He went to the hospital where the neurologist is based and luckily found him there. He signed the death certificate, but it was he who had included the question mark.

We were told the post-mortem would take about six weeks. After five weeks, the neurologist rang to say he wanted to come and tell us the results. He had obviously been told to do this by the CJD Unit in Edinburgh, because an announcement about the new strain CJD, caused apparently by BSE, was being made in the House of Commons by the Secretary of Health the next day.

Martin Zeidler did come down from the CJD Unit in Edinburgh. He told us that the plan had been to inform the relatives of the ten people who had new strain CJD before any public announcement was made. This they had been unable to do because news about the discovery of the new strain and its link with BSE was being announced in the House of Commons by the Secretary of Health.

Had Dr. Narang not diagnosed CJD by his urine test and encouraged me to have that finding confirmed, I would have been less likely to demand the post-mortem which he regarded as essential, if we were ever to know the truth. Had I not insisted on having that, I suspect Peter's death would have been blamed on something other than CJD. Both the urine test and the post-mortem not only confirmed that Peter had, in fact, died from CJD but left the Government with no alternative but to admit that a new strain of CJD had appeared.

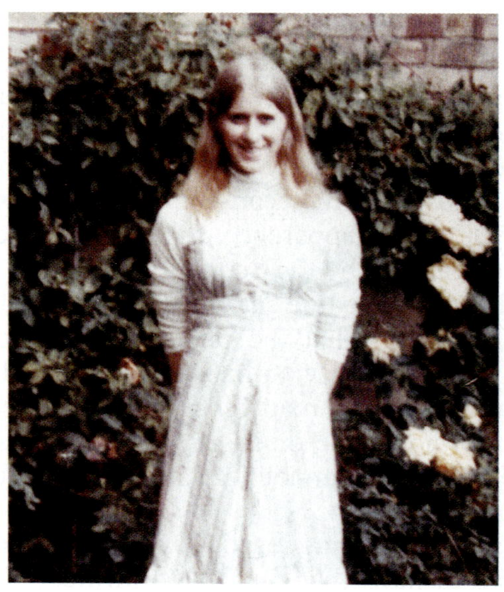

Jean Wake

Jean Wake of Washington, near Sunderland, died in November 1995 from CJD at the age of 38. She was unable to recognise her family for the last three months of her life. Jean was the first person to be diagnosed, while still alive, as having CJD, after her family asked me to conduct my specially-developed urine test. She died shortly after I confirmed that she had CJD. Jean, a divorcee, had a 15-year-old daughter. She bought cheap meat from someone selling it door-to-door.

Jean's 74-year-old mother, Nora Greenhalgh, wrote a series of letters to Government ministers, including Prime Minister John Major, and the Opposition leader, campaigning for recognition of my urine test for CJD.

After Jean's death, she said: "Now that it's finally over, it is a blessing." Here, Nora describes how CJD brought about her daughter's death.

It was about 1988 when Jean's talking started to go funny. She would race on, and I would say: "Jean, take your time. I can't understand what you're talking about." Later on, she slurred her speech. She smoked heavily, and we thought she must be starting to suffer from a stroke. She had difficulty writing. It became worse until she could not write at all. She was a healthy woman apart from that. She was a happy girl and used to turn men's heads. She used to hold herself well.

When she came back from London to live here, she worked in an electrical factory in Washington. Then she did odd jobs, such as selling sandwiches around the factories. But no one would employ her as she became worse. You only had to speak to her to know she was not right.

From 1991, she started falling about and walking with her stomach stuck out. People used to ask whether something was wrong with her spine. She would fall in the bus, and whenever she was outside. I thought her shoes were to blame, and I told her to buy some flat ones. We did not know what on earth was the matter.

She was very aggressive. It was like living on a volcano, you did not know when she was going to explode. She would come in nice as ninepence, then you would say something to her, and she would stand up and yell at you: "I hate you, I hate you." When she had calmed down, she would say: "Mum, I don't hate you." We did not know what to do. At first, we thought she was just having tantrums, but then we realised she was ill. I used to dread her coming over here, because you had to be so careful what you said to her.

She would never tell us what she thought was wrong with her. She would just say that she had to go to the doctor's again, because she had another cold. I told her to tell the doctor everything, and she said she had. He gave her Valium. I phoned the doctor, and said that I was not happy about Jean. He would not talk to me because of patient confidentiality. I phoned my son-in-law, and told him I was worried about her and what people were saying. They were calling her a funny woman.

Then she became worse. In 1993, my son-in-law, arranged for Jean to have a scan. I kept asking her whether she had heard from the hospital. She kept saying that everything was all right. We did not know then that she was taking the post and destroying the letters because they wanted to admit her to hospital.

We had her admitted to hospital and they wanted her to walk. I told them it was cruel because they knew she could not do it. I had a talk with the doctor about a fortnight after she was admitted, and I asked him what he was doing. He said that they did not know what to do. They thought she had Huntington's Chorea. Later, he said it was not that. I told him I had seen a few people die, and I knew that my daughter was dying. He just looked at me. I asked: "Is she dying, doctor?" He did not answer.

We were told that her brain had been shrinking for two years. She was trembling all the time. She could not hold a cup properly. I used to say: "You're worse than me, and I'm old." She gradually became worse and worse, until, one morning she could not hold the cup at all. She could not sit on a chair properly. She could not stand.

Jean gradually grew worse. At the end, you could see her bones. She did not know anyone: she was in a coma. They sedated her for about six weeks before she died. We could see her looking at us and we would say: "Try and squeeze our hand if you know what we are doing," but there was no response. She could not swallow. She kept grabbing her throat, grabbing the tubes. She got her hand round her throat one day, and they had a job getting it loose. They said she was going into little fits.

I asked for her to be sent to Newcastle for tests in July. After only a week in hospital there, she did not recognise us. Dr Martin Zeidler of the CJD Unit in Edinburgh came down and said that he was 98 per cent sure it was CJD and she had not long to live. We arranged for her to be sent back to Sunderland. I had never heard of CJD. I phoned a consultant and he said that it was mad cow disease.

They did blood tests and a doctor come down again specially from the Unit in Edinburgh to see us about this. He tried to tell us that it could be hereditary, that Jean had been born with it. He asked me to have a test done saying I could live till I was 90 year old but still end up with CJD. He said that, if I was positive, it meant that my family had a 50-50 chance of getting it.

If I was negative on the other hand, that meant my husband could have had it, but he's dead, so there's no way of proving that. I wouldn't like to think that he's to be blamed for it. There's no-one on his side and no-one on mine who has had a similar disease. ***Tony, my son, talked about being tested, because he's thinking about starting a family, but I think he's changed his mind and I've changed my mind. I told him: "I***

would willingly have the test but I have a cousin who advised against it". He told me: "You are 77 now. You've gone through enough, live your life out the way it is now".

On that Monday when I saw the "World in Action" about CJD, I decided I should let people know that it was up here. No-one up here knew it was here. I phoned the local evening newspaper, the Sunderland Echo, at 10 pm and asked if they were interested. They said they were, and a reporter came round the next morning.

That was the first reporter. From then it escalated. All the papers came. They were knocking at the door. I never used to get upset when I was being interviewed, but I would cry at night-time. I do not know how I had the strength to go through with it. You know, somehow I felt as though I was being stopped from talking to the papers. ***I felt I was being gagged. I was asked by the hospital who had given the details to the papers and I told them straight out that it was me. I said we'd called Dr Narang in - but the doctor wasn't very pleased. Albert had found out about your urine test for CJD and he phoned me up and said: "I'm going to talk to a Dr Narang and ask him to do this test on our Jean". He did phone the hospital asking them to allow Dr Narang to do the test and give him the specimens. The doctor from the hospital sounded very sweet on the phone but then they put obstacles in our way. He said: "If you want to have a scientist like that in, it's up to you, but you know what some of these scientists are". He rang me up a few times. I don't know why they were going to all this trouble.*** There's something that they are trying to hide, something they are trying to stop me from saying, I don't know what.

She was dead and that was it. Everybody up here was pleased that I had done what I did. It helped to bring it out in the open. People would come up to me in the street and say: "I think you've done the right thing to let everyone know". Even you, Harash, didn't know I was writing to John Major. That was in July. I blame the beef for infecting her and I feel very strongly about it. I have believed all the time that it was the beef, somehow. There is something that they are trying to hide.

Harash: Tell about the chap who used to bring meat around.

Nora: Yes, He used to bring beef, and we used to buy about

20 or 30 lbs of beef steak and mince at just 50p a pound and sometimes I got ox tails. He used to come to our Jean's door in Washington. She used to work as a barmaid and he got on talking to her. I used to get 10 lbs of steak and 10 Ibs of mince a week. That was about 1990. Whether this meat has fallen off the back of a lorry or was from a knacker's yard - from casualty cattle - we never knew. We never asked any questions. She was on income support. She needed to buy cheap meat.

You wanted to know about her teeth. She had pyorrhoea in the gums when she was just 17 or 18 years old and they cut all her gums to get the pyorrhoea out and they capped all her teeth. She was like that till she died.

I wrote two letters to John Major, the Prime Minister, and one to Douglas Hogg, the Agriculture Secretary. In the first one to the Prime Minister, I told him he should tell people the truth, but I never had a satisfactory reply.

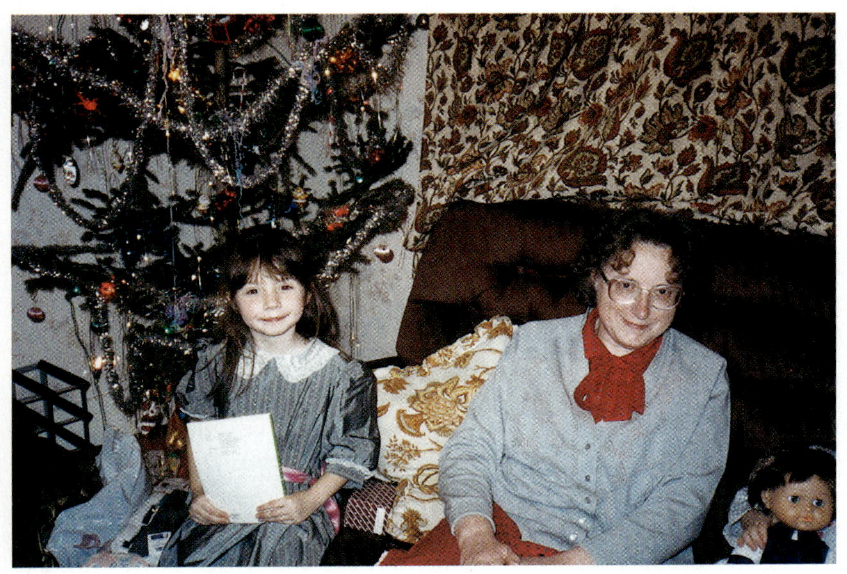

Joan Davidson and Elizabeth Bottle

Margaret Ammon's two younger sisters, twins Joan Davidson and Elizabeth Bottle, both of Ashford, Kent died of CJD. Margaret recalls her thoughts and describes how her sisters developed the clinical symptoms about six years apart. They lived together for 42 years and had only been separated in the past ten years. She and her husband compared the two sisters' clinical symptoms with what they had seen in BSE cows on their farm. Joan Davidson, who died first at the age of 51 in 1989, woke up one morning with her shoulder hurting. Her doctor diagnosed a trapped nerve in her shoulder. Within days, she developed weakness in her legs and found it difficult to walk but she was being treated only for depression. Huntington's Chorea, a hereditary condition, was suspected and that created panic in the family. The fear was that other family members might develop it soon. In Guy's Hospital, after an EEG test was done, her family were told she had CJD. Joan has been a blood donor from 1981 when she got married.

In September 1996, Margaret's second sister, Elizabeth Bottle, after being ill for 18 months, died, at the age of 59. Around 1991, she had had a blood transfusion following an ulcerated gullet. This could be significant as she was living in a high risk area - Ashford, which has had a cluster of CJD cases.

Starting with a slight tremor in her hands, the early symptoms of Parkinson's disease gradually progressed until Elizabeth was staggering and losing her balance and started falling over, just as Joan had done, reminding the family once again of BSE symptoms. Margaret asked Harash to do his live urine test. That was done and Elizabeth was found positive for CJD. The family also discussed the importance of a post-mortem with Harash and asked him to witness the post-mortem and to do other independent necessary tests on her brain.

In the case of Joan, no post-mortem was done. Examination of Elizabeth's brain, however, revealed extensive vacuolation of the cerebellum and numerous PrP positive plaques. These clinical symptoms and pathological changes are typical of Narang disease caused by the BSE strain of agent. It is claimed that this is a disease affecting only the young, the under 40. Elizabeth's case, however, shows that the BSE strain agent affects all age groups.

Here, the family describe their horrific experiences in caring for two victims of CJD and the scar it has left on them for life.

Margaret: Well, I had two sisters Joan and Elizabeth and both ended up much the same way. I was 23 when I got married and I lived at home until then. ***They were three and a half years younger than me. I left home when I got married and they lived together right up until Joan married eight years now. So the three of us had lived together for about 20 years and Joan and Elizabeth continued living together for a total of 42 years, right up until Joan got married in 1981. They both developed CJD.*** Joan was the first to be hit by this dreadful disease. She was only 51. To start with, we did not realise there was much the matter with her. We went down to see her, it would be late 1988, just before Christmas. We went out shopping together. We chatted and she seemed perfectly okay. Her husband was there and he kept having to remind her, "Joan, I told you about so and so". I didn't think of it at the time, but, looking back, that probably was the start of it. Her memory didn't seem to be what it had been.

After that, I didn't see her again until the second week of January. We were going to see my husband's mother and we had a Kentucky down the road. We all sat round with our Kentucky boxes nattering, because my mum was alive at that time, and she was ill, well, she'd got Parkinson's and had that for quite a number of years. I did not see anything wrong or unusual in Joan that worried me. Nothing struck me as being any different from normal. She was just like I am now. As I say, the only thing was she was getting a little bit, just a little bit forgetful.

That was on the Saturday. On the Sunday, Joan rang me up and said: "Oh, Margaret, I feel funny. Well my arm's all gone dead, my left arm".

"What", I said. Have you lain on it awkward or something?"

I could tell she was worried and she told me that she had woken up with it in the night with her fingers feeling like sausages, and her shoulder hurting. I thought she might have had a slight stroke or something during the night and went round the farm to see Derek my husband. He agreed with me and I rang back to speak to her and suggested she should get on to the doctor straight away. Her husband answered the phone and he too had been advising Joan to see the doctor but she wanted to leave that till the next day, just because it was Sunday. We chatted for a few minutes and he finally decided to call the doctor.

Joan's husband rang back about half past twelve to tell me, "The doctor's been in and he said she's got a trapped nerve in her shoulder. He has given her some tablets and says that, if it doesn't get any better, she might have to wear a collar".

So I said: "Oh well that is good. You know at least you have had him out, and it is good to know it is only a trapped nerve. That is not as bad as having a stroke".

When I went to see her she was not shaking in any way. Yes, she did get just a little bit forgetful or confused but that was all at that time. After that Sunday she rang me twice in the week and said: "I am no better and my arm shakes in a strange way. I just cannot stop it shaking. Yes, it keeps doing silly things". So anyway, she went to see the doctor a second time. She phoned me after she has been to see him and he had told her: "You're getting yourself in such a state, Mrs Davidson, that I'm going to give you something to calm you down". So he put her on some tranquilliser.

Richard, her husband, phoned me two days later and said: "She went down to the doctor's, and she was in a terrible state and he said to her "I'll give you some more anti-depressants You're getting yourself into a state about nothing. It's merely a pinched nerve. Go back home. I don't want to see you again until April". On the 18th March she died. That was after her GP had said to her, "I don't want to see you until April". You know, the doctor thought the tablets would do her good. It wasn't only her arms, in fact, her legs had started to go wobbly. She was in a terrible state and having difficulty keeping her balance. I couldn't get her to calm down.

To start with, it was the left arm and then the left leg. She was also getting a bit of pins and needles in both legs and she became very unsteady on her legs. She went back again to see her doctor. This time Richard went with her and he then changed her medication.

A friend of Elizabeth went to see Joan. She really got a fright when she saw her. She could hardly walk round. Her legs were going. It was as though she has got paralysis. Joan had been walking to the doctors, 500 yard from her home, two week before that and now she could not walk 5 yards. I wondered what sort of trapped nerve had she had got which could cause this. Her trouble really was that she just couldn't balance herself.

We drove down about two weeks later to see Joan, she looked, well, 20 years older than when I had last seen her. One arm was just shaking unstoppably while her left leg was doing jerky movements, although not so badly when she was sitting. She couldn't stop them. If she picked anything up it just went out of her hand. She had no power, no grip. She would hold onto furniture on the way round the room, yes exactly like a baby.

I said straight-away, "This is not a trapped nerve. This is serious". She had to hold onto something and sort of walk round it. I felt very angry because I felt the doctor should have known that it was something more than a trapped nerve which the doctor was thinking of treating with steroids. She should have been more aware of "Mad cow disease".

From that day on, we said: "Right we've got to get her to the hospital". The doctor came out and immediately sent her straight to the William Harvey Hospital in Ashford. I said to Derek, "Well now she's there, you'll be able to get something done. At least you'll know something is being done". I think it was four days later they did a brain scan. Obviously she was getting worse all the time.

Well, the doctors thought she had Huntington's Chorea. We were told that was hereditary. She was too young to die. Of course, my immediate reaction was panic. Derek and I went through our family records and we couldn't think of anybody who had it.

When we first picked her up, before she went into William Harvey, she was reading a newspaper when, all of a sudden her arm went out like that and the paper flew, and I said to her, "What did you do that for Joan?" and she said: "Well, I didn't do it on purpose" and I picked it up and gave it back to her. A few minutes later, the same thing happened again.

Joan was moved to Guy's hospital in London and she stayed there for ten days. She'd be talking, like I'm talking now, about things going on around her......being in hospital, hoping they could soon find out what's wrong with her.....How's Richard going to cope while she was in there.... That sort of thing. She'd talk about the people who sent her in flowers and cards although, now and again she would tend to go off track and talk about something else. I could see no signs of dementia. But, by her third day in Guy's, when I saw her, her legs were almost gone. She was shuffling to the toilet with the aid of a nurse. So, in those few days between leaving Ashford and getting to Guy's, her legs had almost gone. She literally was walking with two people keeping her up. I mean, within a fortnight it had progressed so she had a nurse either side of her, one under each arm, her feet would be almost dragging. They'd be almost half carrying her. Her arm had stopped shaking but her legs were just sort of like, spread out. She still laughed. She still could see the funny side of things. She was still talking. She did tell me at that point, "They are going to do a lumbar puncture". She was to have one of those done.

She was in Guy's for ten days. Well, when they had nearly finished all the tests, we went in the following Wednesday, and the doctors called us in and went all through her medical history with us and wanted to know whether she had any other partners. She hadn't. Had Richard had lots of partners? Could there be VD? Could there be any of these sort of things? The only thing we could tell them was that mum had Parkinson's for about 15 years from the start until she died at the age of 85.

The doctor said: "Well, I did say it wasn't going to be good news. "We have had all the tests back and I'm afraid she's got Creutzfeldt-Jakob Disease". He said they'd done an EEG and the brain had already shrunk. Well, at that stage I hadn't ever heard of that disease. I'd heard of Mad Cow disease, because we'd had it on our farm, but I hadn't heard of CJD. I asked the doctor "What is that?" The doctor said: "Well it's a brain disease. It's a virus that we pick up and it affects the brain. There is no treatment. Nothing can be done. She will not recover. She has got three months, six months, maybe a year, at the outside, to live. I would say somewhere nearer three to six months rather than a year". So, when we had finished talking with him, we went off and made ourselves look a bit presentable and everything and, then, we went back to Joan's bedside. She said to Richard, "I wonder how long you'll have to look after me". And he said: "Well, of course I'm going to look after you".

They transferred her back from there to the William Harvey and after that she lived another fortnight. That last week of her life, we really wished ..... you know we were praying ..... that she would go because it was awful, just awful.

Once she was back in Ashford, they put her onto drugs and that helped the shaking. That wasn't so bad, but her jaw wouldn't open. She had lots of jerks. Suddenly it came over her and then she calmed down. If you moved her from one place to the other, then it would become noticeably worse.

You have got to remember that she got worse very rapidly and, apart from the last week, she understood everything you said to her although, at that stage, because of her teeth being jammed together, she had difficulty in saying anything. I suppose a fortnight before she died her speech was beginning to get as though she'd perhaps had a little bit too much to drink. Yes, slurred: that would be a good description. I am sure her mind was okay. It seemed to be that it affected her more in a physical sense than a mental sense.

She was feeding herself to start with but, when she got back to the Harvey, I was feeding her and I had difficulties with the spoon - her teeth would clench if you got the spoon in and you couldn't get it out.

It was different when it came to be Elizabeth's turn. She was different. Joan didn't appear to lose her mental faculties so much as she did her physical ones.

Joan was keen on her cat, always petting it and, of course, she often got scratched. She was always feeding it and, naturally, would have handled cat food. Before she was married she worked in a commercial type of laundry with her twin sister, but, even there, you can't tell what she would have been handling. There could well have been clothes and overalls handed in from the abattoir for cleaning.

They loved lamb, and my mum was the same. Lamb was their main choice... from a local butcher down the road they used to get it. He used to make his own sausages and that sort of thing, yes on the premises. He would have gone out of business by the time that BSE came in. Yes, by then he would have retired. They often used to kill a steer and they used to send that into the local butchers and he used to joint it all up. It wasn't a regular thing, just about once or twice a year, I suppose. We all ate burgers and sausages. They had a lot of pies, you know, pre-packed pies. When they were at the laundry, they had a canteen there and it was subsidised so they got their meals cheaper. They would have the usual sort of things, sausages, burgers, any sort of pies, chicken pies, beef and onion pies. And they used to have minced meat. Shepherds pie.

Harash: Sausages, you know, are safer to eat than burgers. Sausages contain a lot of fat and, when you cook them, the temperature goes well over 120 degrees and that kills the infection. It's not like that when you cook burgers. They get nothing like so hot: they're often eaten only half-cooked.

Margaret: It is possible, as you say, that they got infected between the time that I got married and Joan got married and left home.... so it could have possibly between 1957 and 1981. They could have both gone out for an evening somewhere and eaten the same infected meal.

Derek: Joan had been a blood donor since she got married and, quite possibly, she was donating blood whilst she was actually incubating the disease. At the time, of course, she thought she was doing the right thing. She used to go about once or twice a year. That, to my way of thinking, is another way I think the disease could be passed on to whoever received the blood. It is a sort of cannibalism, isn't it? You weren't eating it, you were having it injected.

Harash: Can I ask you one more question? Was Joan's condition confirmed by examination? Was there a post-mortem?

Margaret: No she didn't have a post mortem.

Derek: Ah well, there was a confusing thing about that, because, although they said she didn't have a post-mortem, when we went to the solicitor and had to produce a copy of the death certificate, Margaret happened to tell him there hadn't been a post mortem and he pointed to the death certificate and told us we were wrong, because there must have been a post mortem to enable them to have put that on the death certificate. They'd put Jakob Disease and pneumonia. So he told us that, although we might not have been told, they must have done one.

Harash: Not necessarily. In those days, they weren't really bothered if it had been clinically diagnosed. They didn't ask you if they could do a post- mortem did they?

They asked Richard and he said: "No".

Harash: So therefore it wasn't done then, with Joan? Can I ask what you plan to have done when it's Elizabeth's turn? Are you going to have a post-mortem done this time?

Yes.

Elizabeth (Betty) Bottle

Margaret: The first thing I noticed with Betty was that her hands had started developing a slight tremor. It wasn't very much to begin with, but you could just see it was there and, later, it became quite a shiver. She knew she was doing it, because she used to try to hide it. Maybe, to begin with, she didn't, because I don't think she realised it when it happened. It was in both her hands and I thought that she'd got the same thing as mum, Parkinson's.

Derek: Well, she did get a bit peculiar. I found that out on one occasion when I asked her a simple thing. I said to her, "Elizabeth, can I have your Ad Scene" because she never read it anyway. That's a free paper that comes through the door. She literally flew off the handle. And I said to Margaret on the way home in the car, "That was an odd reaction from Betty. I only asked her if I could have her Ad Scene". I thought she over-reacted. You'd have thought I'd asked her for a gold mine.

Margaret: That went on for about a year, and she was gradually getting a more and more shaky, and then she started forgetting things. She'd write things on the calendar, things like dentist's and doctor's appointments and then she wouldn't turn up for them because she didn't remember to look on the calendar to see what she had to do. I'd be phoning her in the morning saying, "Oh you've got a dental appointment today, haven't you,Betty?" or whatever. "Oh no, not till next week", she would say. She was getting terribly confused and forgetful. She was also having difficulty keeping her balance. She had several falls and all she could say was, "I don't know how I did it - I just went". I had to walk with her to support her. She had difficulty co-ordinating her feet to go up steps - even three steps.

Her way of walking didn't alter, not as far we could see. Her difficulty seemed to be that, when she had to negotiate steps, she had to have a rail to hold on to and she would go up one step at a time, moving first one foot onto the step and then the other onto the same step. It seemed to be the forward movement with her that was affected more than anything else. Coming down steps, she was just as bad. It was a problem of co-ordination when it came to negotiating steps, either up or down.

She got a bit aggressive too and, on more than one occasion, she slammed the receiver down. She'd forget things, then she'd say: "No, no, this isn't right", or "that's not right", and then, I'd go over several times with her, the things that she had to do. Simple little things they would be, and I'd have to tell her them two or three times, and then she'd relay it back to me two or three times, and then I'd say: "Have you got that?" and then, she'd start all over again. Repeating over and over again what I'd said: as if she couldn't really grasp what I'd told her. That went on for quite a while. She was living by herself at that time.

She was doing all sorts of things on her own. The neighbours actually told us about it all in the end. We didn't realise just how bad she was getting. She would put an egg on and turn the gas on and then forget it. We went round there one day. The stove was a few feet away from her, and she had the gas alight but was standing in the middle of the kitchen with a saucepan in her hand stirring it. We could see she was getting quite bad by then.

That was in the last few months and she came to stay here with us. At Easter time, she was upstairs for about half an hour and I knew she must be dressed, so, I went up and she was still standing there trying to get her buttons done up.

She was admitted to the hospital. We told the hospital doctor about all the peculiar things that had been happening, he merely thought it was because she had lost blood. She had problems losing blood and the doctor knew about this and, in fact, the hospital had been regularly checking on this for some time.

Harash: You were telling me about that bleeding. Could you tell me more about that, what happened and when?

Margaret: In about 1993, we went for coffee to Littlewoods' and she was sitting there and she said to me, "I think I'll have to go to the doctors". So, naturally, I said: "Why, what's wrong Bet?" She said: "I am having awful trouble going to the toilet. I can't pass anything. I am having trouble. I've been taking things and they don't seem to do any good". So I said: "Well, you'd better go then. You'd better make an appointment for Monday". Anyway, off she went on the Monday and I phoned her up and she said: "Oh yes, I've been" and on the Thursday she had a phone call asking her to pack a small case, the bare necessities, toiletries and the like, and get a taxi up to the doctor's for a letter to take to the hospital. He told her she needed some blood because she was anaemic. So, she went to the hospital.

Well, that was about five or six years ago. They found she had an ulcerated oesophagus. She'd actually bled from that so badly that she needed five and a half pints of blood.

We didn't know how she had managed to keep going. She came out of hospital but they kept a close eye on her from then on. She went every month for a while for blood tests. Then it became every three months, then every six months.

Coming back to the present, it wasn't until the shaking started and then got worse and worse that we began to worry. She came up here at Christmas and she wasn't too good. After some six month without it getting better, we noticed that her co-ordination wasn't quite right and we got her to the doctor's. By then, we'd been saying to the doctors at the hospital that she wasn't right, that she was getting forgetful.

Harash: Was that the same doctors you had seen before? The same doctors you had seen when you were at the hospital with Joan?

Margaret: The GP was exactly the same, but the Doctors at the William Harvey weren't always the same.

Harash: Did he know the situation and what had happened to your other sister?

Margaret: Oh, yes, the G.P. knew that Joan had died of CJD, yes. His receptionist, in actual fact, was saying how unwell she was, but all he was saying all the time was that there was nothing wrong with her. The receptionist was making a better diagnosis than he was. When Betty was eventually taken into hospital this time, I went down with her and she was taken into the emergency ward. They were going to send her home but I refused to let her come out. I said: "Well you sign me a piece of paper to say she can go home on her own, because I'm not taking that responsibility". The doctor had sent her in so that she could be admitted. There was quite a commotion then. I had quite a scene with the medical staff. They kept her in on that Saturday night and then said they had completed the blood tests and she could go home. She was all right, they said.

When I went to her doctor the following Monday, he was on holiday and another chap was there in his place. He said the doctor was treating her for anaemia. I said: "Why are they treating her for anaemia? She's been going to the hospital for three years, and now you're telling me he's treating her for anaemia. Either you're wasting my time, or I'm wasting yours. I've got a lot more things to do that are more important", and with that, I walked out. I was furious. All the nurses in the clinic had been saying for the last year "Doesn't Betty look ill. I wonder what's wrong with her?" She'd lost two and a half stones in weight. They knew the whole story, all the details. They'd been told: "She's losing weight, she's not remembering things, she's having falls". They'd been told it all, but not one of them picked it up, or had her in for observation. That Saturday, when she went to the hospital and I had refused to take her out, she was seen in the casualty ward. On the Sunday they transferred her to the gynaecology ward, because they hadn't got a bed anywhere else. She stayed there until she went to Guy's four days later.

Harash: Why did they send her to Guy's?

Margaret: Because I had told them that her sister had died from CJD, and she was now losing weight and I was worried about her. They were concerned also because she couldn't even lift her arms up. She couldn't stand. She had aged very considerably, and she looked about 80. They realised there was something seriously wrong. She was claiming that a spirit was following her around.

Derek: She thought someone kept poking her in the back. Hallucinations. That's what it was She was absolutely petrified.

Margaret: One afternoon, about Easter, 1995, she took herself to the solicitors in Ashford and made a will. She left there - we presume she went home - but at 9 o'clock that night, she turned up at a friend's home about four or five miles away, to ask him if he would do the hymns for her funeral. She had written in her will what she wanted done with her possessions, with the various things that she had. The only thing that she got wrong was what she wanted to leave to her three cousins. It may seem funny, but she wanted to leave £15 to each of them so that they should buy flowers. That was the only peculiar thing. She wasn't in a confused state. She said to me: "You've got to get things right, because, if anything ever happens, you've got to be sure that everybody is going to get what you wanted them to have". From that day on, she went downhill. She thought she had Parkinson's.

Harash: So, when she was transferred to Guy's, what happened then?

Margaret: She was at Guy's for a month and they did all sorts of tests. They took her to Queen Mary's at Paddington for more tests and yet more at another hospital. Then they sent her back to the William Harvey, but, obviously, they couldn't keep her there long-term, because it was a major hospital, so they transferred her to the Ashford British Geriatric. She was under the same consultant as had attended her sister. They'd been through all Joan's medical records as well. Dr Colchester, it was. A very, very nice man. She went back to Guy's in the November for another ten days where they did some more scans, but there were no changes for either the better or the worse. When she was back at Ashford, he came to see her on 6th February, and they took her over by ambulance to the Harvey. We went over there to see him, and Betty was in a pretty bad state by then. He said that she was to remain in hospital and told us she might have another two or three months, that was all. That was in February. Dr Colchester told us then what her trouble was. She had CJD and he stressed to us that it could be genetic.

By then, she had very starey eyes. She got those jerks. All of a sudden, she'd shiver. You could see the body shaking as well. They stepped up the medication she was getting, that's all they were doing. If I went up behind her, and she didn't realise I was there and I just tapped her on the shoulder, you'd think she'd had an electric shock the way she jumped.

Her speech was slurred, but she was also having a job connecting her brain to what she wanted to say and she'd go on for hours and hours. She could not get the words out, there was more to it than just slurring Sometimes, she would focus on just one thing - often it was me - and ignore everything else going on around her. Even when you called her name quite loudly several times and touched her and said: "Listen, I'm trying to tell you something", it didn't seem to connect. Her eyes were open wide and she'd just go on with what she had been saying. You just weren't getting through to her.

I feed her quite often when I go. She was finding swallowing difficult, sometimes it doesn't always go down. If you are giving her liquids she'd take it in and then, it would start coming back out of her mouth rather than going back down. They were saying before the last time I went to see her that they might have to put a drip in, but I have stipulated that I don't want her force fed. I don't really see any point in force feeding her.

Harash: Some people have a lot of saliva and have difficulty swallowing it. And then, people get worried that they'll get contaminated wiping it away and so on.

Margaret: She did have a spell when she brought up rather a lot of liquid like .... a whole lot came out all at once. The last time I was down on the Wednesday, Friday and Saturday, she was bringing up a lot of .. black, it was, and that is when they said they would probably have to put her on a drip. I'll go down again tomorrow. I haven't rung today because I was told not to ring.

Harash: It's a very difficult situation. We have already talked about what she ate and the two of them, Betty and Joan, lived together so, whatever they did eat it would be the same for them both. You mentioned David Churchill before. How did you know about him?

Margaret: I knew that David Churchill had lost his son, and I knew the area around Devizes where he came from, so, I got his number and got in touch with him.

Harash: The reason I ask is this. Stephen used to have holidays as a boy on a farm near Ashford, and I know he was injured when he was there. It would be interesting if everything could be linked to the one farm. Barbara, who also died of CJD, although living in Luton when she died, did live in a tied cottage on a farm near Ashford for a number of years.

Margaret: I can see the point you are making and the reason why you are interested.

Harash: I know from the urine test that Betty has CJD and nothing is going to save her but I do feel that it will do a lot to help for the future to have it confirmed by post-mortem and I hope you agree.

Margaret: We will certainly ask for a post- mortem and send a letter asking you to be present.

Harash: I think that would be the best thing to do. A final

thought that crosses my mind is that Betty did receive a fairly large volume of blood over the last four years while Joan was a blood donor. Joan, of course, died before Betty started needing transfusions. They both, however, did have connections with the Transfusion Service. We do know that when laboratory animals are injected with blood from CJD patients, they develop the disease. With the known high prevalence of CJD in the Ashford region, it may well be that Joan was not the only donor to be afflicted with CJD. It may well be that Betty got her infection through a blood transfusion, a possibility that surely merits thorough investigation. It certainly would be of interest to know the medical histories of the donors who contributed the blood Betty received.

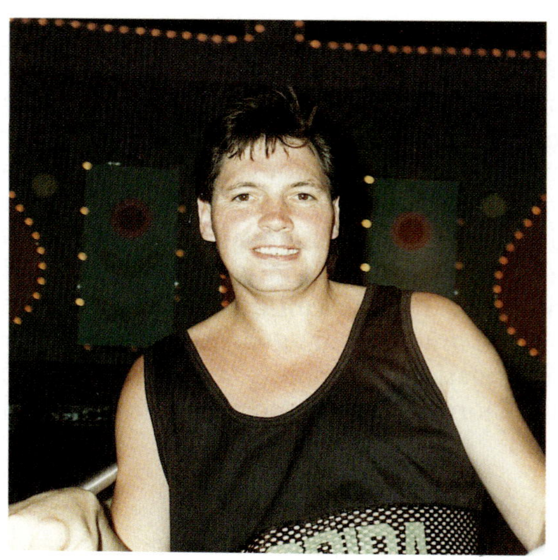

Keith Humphrey

Keith, at the age of 41, became ill and his wife Carol describes in May 1996, how he changed dramatically from being the sociable fun-loving person she had known from childhood and how, from the start of his illness she had nursed him at home. She talked of all the difficulties that this involved as his illness progressed, how his increasing staggering and difficulty in walking necessitated the transfer of his bed to the ground floor when he could no longer climb the stairs. His outings became more and more rare as CJD got the upper hand. Carol, leaving Keith with a friend looking after him, joined Harash in the kitchen where she could feel free to talk. There she outlined her experiences and described the typical symptoms of Narang disease: depression, staggering, falling over, having difficulty in walking. Initially, he was sensitive to his tendency to stagger and, when out, used a walking stick to let other people know that he was not drunk. He had been a regular blood-donor and the final occasion on which he had donated blood was only some six months before the appearance of his symptoms. Carol tells of all the frustrations she had to endure and the scar the disease is going to leave on her and, as a nurse herself continuously nursing a victim of CJD, of the tremendous pressure placed on any family it hits.

Keith's wife telling the story while he has been ill for 9 months (14 Dec 1996 Keith is still alive)

Shall I tell you a little bit about Keith first? He is 41 years old and he's a diesel fitter. He worked for the local bus company. Usually, he's a very jovial outgoing person, and always the life and soul of the party. We enjoyed a busy social life. We were out four or five nights a week, either socialising with friends or just together. He enjoyed crown green bowls which he's played for about ten or twelve years. All in all, a very active sort of person. Very active in his mind as well. He enjoyed quizzes. He was very good at remembering information and the general knowledge type of information. Very quick-witted.

We had known each other since 1974 and we got married in 1984. We lived together for four years before that, so we've actually between together for 16 years and going out together for 22 years, since Keith was about 18. The first signs that anything was slightly amiss was just forgetfulness and that really began at the end of 1994, beginning of 1995. The sort of things that he'd do was he'd double-book events with friends and family. If we were out, and he had to go and get a round of drinks, he'd forget what people had and that might only be say in a group of four of us but it was becoming obvious to me and our friends.

Yes, it became a bit of a joke, because Keith was 40, 18 months ago, and he just put it down to the fact that, "I'm 40 now, and getting on a bit, you've got to expect these things to start happening." We've got a friend who is forgetful by nature and we used to compare him with Keith and say: "You're getting more and more like Andy."

He's always been a very humorous person. I noticed last year that sometimes he started to overstep the social boundaries with his humour. It just wasn't acceptable, I felt, although none of our friends were concerned. They'd always joked with him because he was always a very straightforward, up-front person. You could say what you wanted to him.

The other thing that he became preoccupied with dying and would always be talking about it. He felt that, because his father had died suddenly at the end of 1993 with a heart attack, he was going to die before he was 62. He'd got shared ownership in the company he worked for and he was holding onto the shares because he felt that they would give him a nest-egg so that he could retire at 50. He was convinced that he was going to die.

Harash: What about his other family, his grandparents?

Carol: All of his grandparents are dead. I think they all lived to fair ages. His grandmother definitely was 84 when she died. His dad's brother died young, in his late fifties, with a heart attack. Over the next few weeks Keith really got worse and the time came when he wouldn't remember conversations. If we'd been out for the evening, the next day I'd say to him, "Well, last night we were talking about that", but he wouldn't remember the conversation. He wouldn't remember the arrangements that we'd made. Obviously he was drinking, so I'd think, well he did have a drink and that was the excuse I made for him not remembering. On average, he'd have about 5 pints, he rarely drank spirits. It got to the stage where he couldn't remember conversations he'd had some hours before. Often he'd think that he'd told me things when he hadn't. He'd say to me, "I've told you that" but I'd have no recollection of it and it would be news to me. He also seemed to drink more alcohol than he had done, more than he was accustomed to drink and more than his friends. He would be "overtaking" whereas, at one time, that wouldn't have happened. He'd be getting up to have a drink, when his friends would still have drinks standing on the table from previous rounds.

Between about the middle of 1995 or possibly about October, his appetite seemed to fall and he lost about a stone in weight and, about the same time, his sex drive decreased. He became depressed and sad. He used to say to me that he was worried, for no good reason I could see and, from what he told me, for no good reason that he could see. He said: "I didn't really have any thoughts or anything in my head and I wasn't thinking about anything in particular but that this feeling just came over me and I just felt as if I wanted to cry". He'd say to me, "I just feel as if I want to cry" and told me that he had felt like that at work sometimes. A couple of times, when I was with him, he would actually cry, but for no reason he could explain. He just didn't know why. He said: "Why am I feeling like this?" That worried him as did the fact that he was losing his sense of humour.

To begin with, Keith was denying that there was anything

wrong with him and claiming that he was upset only by the deaths of a few of our friends but, in October 1995, I finally persuaded him to go and see his GP. We went and saw our GP and he diagnosed clinical depression and Keith was put on some anti-depressants.

Harash: Did ever he mention that he felt empty, that he had nothing in his mind, nothing in his brain?

Carol: Later on he did but not at that time. I don't recall him saying anything to me like that at that time but it certainly happened later on. As things got worse he couldn't find the words he wanted to use, but was much later on.

About that time, he used to take very personally any news of disasters or anything sad on television as if it was a personal disaster to him and became very disturbed and frightened.

In November 1995, after Keith started the anti-depressants he did feel better in himself, and actually was promoted at work. He had been working towards that for a long time and it did seem to buck him up and make him seem a lot better although he was still as forgetful. His sleep pattern changed from that time. He used to fall asleep a lot when he came home from work, and that wasn't like him. He'd always had great difficulty in sleeping. From then on, he'd fall asleep in his chair and he started to going to bed early as well. Another thing I noticed was that, from about this time, he started repeating himself a lot during.

Then, round about December 1995, he began to lose his co-ordination and started being very clumsy with food. If he was eating, he'd spill it or he'd drop it. He developed a tremor as well. He became very restless, very fidgety, couldn't keep still, was always crossing and uncrossing his legs and moving his position in the chair. He was getting clumsy. He would say: "Oh look I'm doing it again." He would get annoyed with himself. He just didn't know why. It seemed to me almost as if he had forgotten that he had something in his hand and he would drop it, a cup or something like that. He'd be talking to you with a drink in his hand and while he was talking to you, you would see he would turn the cup over.

We went away for the new year, and we stayed in the same hotel we had been to every year. He couldn't remember the room number or where the room was situated in the hotel and this in the hotel we had been to every year for the last 8 years. He did remember the proprietor of the hotel and other people we knew, but wouldn't remember the names of any new people we met at this time. He seemed to drink an awful lot alcohol whilst we were away. It was really his short-term memory that was worst. He couldn't remember what the GP said to him, and he forgot the advice he had been given. He forgot his anti-depressants when we went away and his mood did seem to plummet towards the end of the five days we were there. He was also falling over things whilst we were there and seemed clumsier than before. I did notice that, sometimes when he was going off to sleep, I thought he was scratching. In fact, I think he was shaking. His hands and arms were shaking, and I would say to him, "Keith are you alright? what are you doing?" He would say "what?" as if he didn't know what I meant. I would say "You were shaking." He would reply, "I'm alright."

When we got back from being away for the New Year in January 1996, we actually went back to the GP to tell him about the tremors. The GP thought it was a side-effect of the anti-depressants and he changed his prescription to Prozac. On that occasion, Keith left the doctor in no doubt as to how badly upset he was. He kept telling the GP how frightened he was that he was going mad, and the GP tried to reassure him that, as he was so aware of what was happening, he, therefore, wasn't going mad. The GP also advised him "to cut your alcohol intake to one pint a day." but Keith immediately forgot what the GP had told him. He had to keep checking with me. How much did he say I could drink? When have I got to go and see him again? He also used to misplace articles. For instance he'd leave his wallet at work: he lost his keys. He was still losing weight and he'd lost about two stone in all by this time.

In mid-February, we went to visit some friends in Scarborough and,by then,he was very clumsy with his food. He was spilling almost everything that he had. He kept repeating himself and was very upset at not being able to drink and he kept blaming me. He really kept going on at me saying that it was because of what I'd done and that it was only me who thought he shouldn't drink alcohol. It wasn't the doctor at all. He thought the doctor hadn't said that. He just wouldn't understand any reasoning.

There was just no reasoning with him.

By February 1996, it was affecting his driving. It was really quite jerky and he sometimes had difficulty changing gears and tended to crash them. He would overreact to things on the road. If somebody was pulling out he would swerve sharply, when actually there was no need for that. While we were away, he actually took a friend out for a drive and she noticed it and commented on his erratic driving and that worried him.

Whenever you asked him how he was, he'd always say: "I'm much better now, much better", and he also kept saying "I've got my sense of humour back now". It seemed he always wanted to reassure himself.

On the way back home from Scarborough, he was very upset about his clumsiness and he cried in the car on the way home. About this time, I noticed that he had difficulty getting in and out of the car. If he was trying to get into it, he would sometimes stand for a few seconds as though trying to think how to put his leg into the car and then how to put the seat belt on. Sometimes he would only put it half way across and not continue to clip it in. If I said to him "Can you put your seat belt on?", he would say: "I know, I know, I'm just doing it." He would get quite angry with me about it. He said that he felt no one would want him around if he was going to be like this. It was very obvious that I was worried sick about what was happening to him. I kept saying to him, "How are you getting on at work. Has anybody noticed anything at work?" All that he could say to me was that his mood was different. Keith felt he was being very unsociable and that people were noticing it. Actually, they were. He was getting really worried by the fact that he was spilling his food on people's furniture and carpets and things like that and it really upset him. He would be over-apologetic and would want me to apologise as well and he found it all very distressing. I mean I myself was worried sick, and I was frightened by how he might be performing at work, because that involved his driving, test-driving buses. I was worried that, in his condition, perhaps he didn't have the skills needed to be able to do that type of work.

I asked him had anyone noticed anything about his work and he kept saying to me that he was fine, because, when he was at work, his mind was occupied and he was fine. I thought and told him, he was getting to the stage where he was actually unsafe, but he kept refusing to believe that. He wasn't the same old Keith. People used to say "What's wrong with you, you're quiet?". But he said that his work itself was fine. I felt that in actual fact he didn't know whether he was safe or not because, although my friends told him that his driving was dangerous, and he did acknowledge it at the time, afterwards he would say: "I'm alright, it's okay". He couldn't see at all that he was ill at that point. When you asked him, he would tell you he was 100%. He wasn't. He was far from it. No-one at work actually mentioned it or made any complaint, but they must have noticed it. He, himself, couldn't actually see, in fact, didn't have any idea at all about how ill he was. On Tuesday, 20th February 1996 which was immediately after the weekend we had been away, he came home from work and said that he'd had a very frightening experience at work. He had to test drive buses as part of his job and, what he'd done was he'd taken the bus out to pick up some equipment from another garage and, on the way there, his mind had just gone blank and he couldn't remember how to get from where he then was to where he was going and he said he had to just stop the bus and sit there until it actually came back to him where he was going and, once he remembered, then he went on to the garage he was going to but, when he arrived, he was too late to pick up the equipment because the stores had closed. He was late getting back to work and they wanted to know where he had been. Luckily it had been snowing and so he said it was the snow which had held him up.

Then on the next night, Wednesday, 21st February - he usually gets home at about 4.45 in the evening and, if he is going to be late, he always rings me - it got to half past five and there was no sign of him. I was very scared stiff and I thought "What's happened, is he stuck somewhere! Does he not know where he is". I tried to ring the garage and eventually, after much ringing, he eventually came home at 7 o'clock. He had no idea of the time and he said that he had lost his keys and that he was looking for them to lock his locker at work. He just couldn't understand why I was upset by his not having come home at the usual time. I was extremely worried by then and I decided to go and see my GP on my own. The very next morning on Thursday,

22nd February, I went to see him and he said he'd see Keith that night. After examining him, he bluntly told Keith that he was unfit to work and unfit to drive and he was going to have further investigations done to see what was wrong with him. He arranged for a psychiatrist to come and do a domiciliary visit the next day, at home. Keith was very frightened when the psychiatrist came and he asked: "Do you think I've got Alzheimer's Disease?" he doctor said: "We can't rule that out" but that, as far as she could see, he didn't have a psychiatric problem, and that he should be referred to a neurologist.

On 28th February, we went to see a neurologist. He examined Keith and said that he didn't think he'd got a brain tumour which had been one of my worries. He took some blood from him and said that he'd arrange for Keith to have a scan and an EEG and Keith was then admitted to the Day Unit. He said that it would take some 8 weeks to set up the tests. I just couldn't see why we should have to wait eight weeks when Keith seemed so acutely ill. Surely, they could have done the tests straight away and got the results almost immediately. His speech was becoming hesitant and some of his speech movements were far from smooth, they were quite jerky. He was really quite unable to understand what was going on around him and why. He was angry with the doctors for not giving him any answers or telling him why he was ill although, all the time, he was still denying that he was really ill.

Keith was definitely preoccupied with going back to work and kept saying that he was determined to go back to work. He'd say to me, "Right that's it, I'm going back to work on Monday" and wouldn't listen to any reasoning about it. Then the day after he said that, on 10 March, he was extremely agitated. He wanted to drive the car. He kept saying: "I am going to drive the car. Why are you trying to stop me? I'll be okay". He kept pacing up and down the room saying that he was going out in spite of his having terrible shakes and jerks.

Harsh: Did the Psychiatrist and the neurologist see those jerky movements?

Carol: Yes, she did. Keith was really very unhappy and down and he kept asking me, "What do they want me to do? When have I got to go again to see them?" For the rest of that week, it was just a case of keeping Keith occupied with work, although, by now I felt that he wouldn't actually know where he was going if he went out. He wouldn't listen to me and I kept trying to come up with a compromise saying: "I'll ring your friend and he'll take you, or else, let me take you". He didn't want to know and kept saying to me he didn't know what I was on about. There was nothing wrong with him. He got furious with me at one point and made me sit down and he just kept repeating the same statements over and over again. He kept saying: "I know what I'm doing. I don't need you or anyone else to tell me. I know what's going on". Some friends came for lunch and I can only describe him as being almost manic in his behaviour, in his expressions, both verbally and facially. They were very exaggerated, very hyper.

There were a few friends who didn't know that he was poorly at that time, and he kept saying: "Don't tell them". On one evening, we were getting ready to go out and Keith was saying something about wanting to go out and have a good drink. I reminded him that the doctor said he could only have a limited amount. I don't quite know why; he just suddenly went berserk, furious and shouting: "I'm not listening to you, you don't know what you're talking about, they don't know what they are on about, nobody can give me any answers".

It was at this point that he kept asking me repeatedly to promise not to tell anyone about his illness and, in particular, not his Mum, because he was concerned about worrying her. I thought that, perhaps when he had calmed down, it would be a good idea to get her to come for a drink with us, which she often did, so I went to the phone. I said to him, "Oh, I'll ask your Mum". I was just trying to say it as casually as possible. "Oh, I'll ask your Mum if she wants to come with us." I was ringing her up to ask her if she wanted to come out for a drink with us when he just suddenly came running down the stairs and ripped the phone off the wall. He was shouting at me that I shouldn't bother an old woman with his problems. He just went absolutely mad and that was completely out of character for him because he was normally very placid. He said: " he was angry because I was ringing his Mum." I think it was because he thought I was going to tell her about his illness although he had already told her himself. She already knew all about it.

Because of the state he was in, I was frightened of him hurting himself and I rang the GP and an on-call doctor came to see him. Keith was very distressed, but he did seem to settle down when that doctor came, and Keith just talked to him very lucidly, telling him that he was fed up about all the tests he was having and he wanted to know what was happening to him. He just didn't understand and he wanted to know. Because she'd heard all the commotion on the phone, his mum actually came round to the house. He wasn't at all bothered by the doctor being there and he calmed down quite quickly at that point.

On 4th March, the Monday, the GP rang the Neurologist to try to get him to hurry up saying we needed the CT scan sorted out quickly. Keith had the CT scan done the following day and the result was negative. That upset Keith again when no cause was found. He kept saying: "I feel fine".

On Wednesday 6th March, the GP came to see him and we had a long conversation about the results of the CT scan and he told me that Alzheimer's hadn't been ruled out. When the GP had gone, Keith wanted me to tell him what had been said. What had happened was this... Keith had gone to put the cats out and, while he was out of the room, I said to the GP, "Keith mentioned to you Alzheimer's. Are we still looking at dementia type illnesses?" The doctor said to me, "Yes it looks increasingly as though that's what it's going to be". Keith had made me promise him that I would tell him everything the medical staff told me without telling him. Keith asked me, "Did the doctor say anything to you when I was out of the room". He wanted to know all that had been said.

I said to Keith, "The doctor told me that they hadn't yet ruled anything out, but it's beginning to look something like Alzheimer's". At that, he just went to pieces and said: "If that's what it's going to be, I just don't want to know". That's just what I expected his reaction to be and why I had been a bit reluctant to tell him. He was very upset, very distressed indeed. We both were and we both cried about it. He went out for a drink with one of his friends, just as they had arranged earlier. He had about two and a half pints of lager and he spilled half of one pint. That really upset and affected him. He seemed to be almost drunk.

That night in bed he was extremely restless. He just kept trying to rearrange his pillows. He kept getting up out of the bed and back again. He just couldn't seem to settle. I tried to cuddle him to try to calm him down and soothe him. I tried to stroke his back and do the things that would normally calm him down. He eventually went to sleep.

By now, his speech was getting worse. He couldn't get the words he wanted out. He would just say half sentences. Like he would start of by saying: "When doctor comes what is it I need to ask him... I've got to ask him about... you know all he would say is b,b,b." He could not complete the word. What he used to do then was try to say things to me. He would be talking to me and all of sudden he would forget what he was trying to say. He would use the wrong words and would say something in a sentence that just wasn't the right word. Something completely out of context. I would laugh at him, we would both laugh and he would try to change it. You probably noticed it yourself. He's always doing it, he realises what he's done, he just laughs.

He also started having difficulty with electrical things, things like the remote control for the television. He'd just sit there with it in his hand and would start doing something with it and, all of a sudden, would stop, and not know what he was trying to do. He bought a new video recorder, but he couldn't see how to set it up and that's the kind of thing he was always good at. One particular morning, he spent an hour just readjusting the position of the television and video.

His appetite at this stage was very poor and he was very concerned about the amount of weight he was losing. If you asked him if he wanted something to eat, he would always say: "No" and yet he was obsessed with the weight that he'd lost.

I'm a nurse and I really harassed a few people to get on and have these tests done because I couldn't wait eight weeks. I rang up one friend and asked if she could sort this EEG out for us and she managed to get it done that same week and on Thursday, 8th March, he had an EEG done. The results were negative, or, at least, we were told no abnormalities were shown.

The week commencing the 12th March, he kept going on about wanting to go back to work and wanting to drive the car. He said he was sure he could drive if I would just gave him a chance. If he couldn't, he agreed he would accept that what I was telling him was right. I did let him drive the car, because I felt, if I let him drive, then he might see how poorly he was driving. In actual fact he felt he'd driven the car quite well when, in fact he hadn't: his driving was quite erratic, all over the place, and yet, he really didn't realise it.

The week commencing the 18th March ,we went to see the same psychiatrist in the Out-patients Department and she asked him how he was? Even though he couldn't speak to her, he managed to say: "The... the..., 100%." His speech was very slurred and he was unable to get the words out. The psychiatrist could see how unsteady Keith was on his feet and the difficulty he had in standing. His balance wasn't quite right. If you didn't know, you'd think he was drunk. When we went to our local pub, people did think he was drunk and that was even before he had had a drink. He seemed to come and go. You would be talking to him one minute and having a conversation and he would be with you for a while, and then someone else might speak and he would be lost. I would say: "Are you listening?", but he just wouldn't be with you for a while, sort of blank.

At that time, we occasionally went out walking, just to pass time. We went for a walk on one occasion to our local shop, and when we came back I deliberately didn't cross the road to where we live. Keith didn't seem to realise quite where we were and made no move to cross. I said: "Keith that's where our house is", and he said: "I know", but I don't think he really did. He would get quite angry about that. The same kind of thing happened at out local shopping centre. He just walked off in the opposite direction to where we were going. To begin with, he would happily manage to walk about quarter of a mile.

At this point he was able to wash and dress, eat and drink himself and go to the toilet independently, but he would take ages to undress, especially at night time. He would repeat his actions, he would undo the belt on his trousers, then he would do it up again and then he would undo it again. He would take his trousers down then pull his trousers up and fasten them back up again. He would keep doing that and it could take an hour for him to get undressed for bed. He would take his trousers off, and I would do everything to encourage him to get undressed but it was difficult. He would go to the toilet and undress himself there for no apparent reason. After a while, I would go to him and say: "You've been in here twenty minutes. Are you okay?" and I'd find him sitting there on the toilet with nothing on at all. He didn't seem to know what he was doing or what he had done, and yet, he wasn't really aware that he had a problem. He would take a lot of coaxing to come back out of the toilet. He would get angry if I tried to explain what he needed to do. "I know, I know" he would say to me and get quite angry with me.

The following day Tuesday 19th March, we had an appointment to go back and see the Neurologist again at the day unit. He told us that, so far, none of the tests they had done showed anything positive and that he could only, "feel that it was some kind of dementia illness". He arranged for Keith to have a MRI scan which, we were told, might mean a wait of several weeks.

After we had seen the neurologist Keith was very upset again to have been given no real answers to his trouble. At that time, his speech was very poor. He could only put a few words together, and he just couldn't really understand what was going on around him. He kept asking me what the doctor had said and when we were to see him again. He was angry and frustrated with everything that evening. Suddenly, at 9 o'clock, as we were sitting watching the television, he leapt up off the settee and, although he was stumbling badly, he just started picking things off the shelves and walking round and round the room and then through the house. He just didn't seem to know what to do with himself. He put soap on his face but didn't know how to get it back off again. I have to give him quite a bit of help and prompt him to get himself washed. I asked him, "What are you doing Keith? What do you want?" He just looked at me staring blankly. I tried to get him to calm down because he was very agitated but he just kept looking at me. He started shouting at me, "Get off" and got increasingly agitated when I asked him what he was trying to do. He said: " I want to go home". He was putting his things together to go home.

He didn't appear to know me at all. Suddenly he got furious and locked himself in the downstairs toilet. He was shouting and banging and I called the GP. He arrived about quarter past ten, and I had to talk to Keith through the toilet door to tell him that the doctor was here to see him. Keith did eventually come out and, although he had met him a couple of times before, he denied knowing the doctor. Keith looked extremely frightened and very pale and was sweating profusely. His eyes were wide open and sort of fixed and staring, and then he just sort of shouted at him, "I don't know you."

Then he went back into the toilet and locked the door behind him. The GP sat with me until about midnight and we could hear Keith banging and muttering away to himself. He eventually came out at about half past one in the morning and he seemed to recognise me then and he put his arms round me and was trying to say something to me, but I couldn't actually make out what. There's a mirror in the toilet and he kept looking into it and laughing as though he was seeing someone else.

The GP gave him some Valium and finally got him to bed about 3 o'clock in the morning. The next day Keith just wouldn't get out of bed: he just stayed there. He refused to have anything to eat or drink. He didn't recognise me at all. I kept going up and down stairs and asking him whether there was anything he wanted, anything he wanted to drink, but he just didn't want anything. I just left the television on for him. I sat with him and slept with him for a little while. I told him, "If there is anything you want, just let me know, and I'll get it for you." He said to me, "But I can't." I said: "Why not?" He said: "Don't you know?" I said: "No. What?" He said: "Because I'm married." It's obvious that he didn't recognise me. He thought I was someone else, but, the next day, he did seem to know who I was. I was able to get him in and out of the bath, and get him dressed.

When he was eating, if I put a sandwich in front of him, or asked him if he wanted something to eat, he would say: "No", so, I started to just give him food, because I don't really think he knew what he was saying. If I put a sandwich in front of him, he could just about manage to eat it. When it came to eating a meal on a plate he just couldn't manage. He couldn't co-ordinate the fork into his mouth and he would drop the food before the food got to his mouth. Sometimes it would go in the wrong direction. So I started to help him to eat and, for a while, he seemed to recognise everyone. The GP came that night and he recognised him.

Over that weekend, the 22nd to 24th March, he got to the stage when he didn't actually recognise the toilet. He got the sensation that he wanted to pass urine, and he would get very agitated and would keep pulling at his trousers or patting his tummy and would be going, "Quick, quick, I want to go." But when I took him to the toilet, he would go, "No, no, no." He just didn't realised what I was trying to do he was incontinent, because we couldn't do anything. I rang the GP on the Monday morning and told him what happened over that weekend. I said I really felt that we had to get him into hospital, and the doctor arranged for him to be admitted to the Neurology Unit at the General hospital.

When he was admitted into the hospital, he could say one or two words - he would say "I know" or he would say: "get off" in a jovial sense. He was laughing all the time and making sounds, saying: "b,b,b,b,.... a lot." You can see him laughing now. He was very alert. Very aware of what was going on around him.

He would mimic facial expressions and the nurses told me that he was normally quite jovial, mimicking me whenever I came into the room. He seemed to understand when I asked him where he was, saying: "I know, I'm in hospital" If his Mum said to him, "This is Carol", he would say: "I know, I know."

He could walk with a little assistance: he really needed guidance. He would eat everything that was offered to him. What did develop was that he was easily startled. If you moved too quickly towards him he would jump. If I went to kiss him on the lips, he would pucker his lips up ready to kiss me but, at the last minute, he would turn his face to one side and I would end up having to kiss him on the chin. He was very keen on watching television and attentive in watching programmes, particularly those he had most enjoyed in the past and which were his favourites and I used to borrow videos of his favourite comedy shows for him and he would watch them and react normally: he would laugh at them and that sort of thing.

He was in hospital for four weeks until he was discharged on Tuesday, 23rd April. By that time his speech had deteriorated to the stage that he would only really say: "hello" or "goodbye", and even that required a lot of prompting. He would repeat whatever you said. He understood commands. If you said:

"Drink this", or "stand", or "look", he would understand that. He only recognised close friends and family. But he also recognised the different doctors and nurses and he would react differently to each one.

He needed a lot of help when it came to standing up and would keep grabbing at things when you were trying to sit him down or stand him up. Very unsteady on his feet, he was, sometimes we would actually need two people to support him when he was walking. He started to drag his right foot at that point. At one time, I could walk him on his own the length of the hospital corridor and that was quite a distance, but what he could do one day would be beyond him the next.

It seemed that he really wanted to eat sweet things like desserts rather than anything else, and he was still drinking very well although, very occasionally, he would pouch food. When he wanted to go to the loo, I would know because he would start fidgeting. His concentration span by then was very poor and he didn't pay much attention to the television at all. But he seemed to enjoy listening to music, so I would play music to him and he tried to... well, he sort of would make noises to it, as if he was trying to sing to it. I felt there was changes in his perception, because, if we were walking down the corridor, he would duck under the door frame as if it was a fright or the space was too small for him to go through. It was the same as we've seen with BSE cows. It was much the same if the television was on and, say a car was speeding towards the screen, he'd try to move out of the way as if it was coming towards him. His sleeping pattern was disturbed as well. Some nights he would lie awake most of the night and then, some days. he would sleep two or three hours at a stretch during the day.

So, looking at the months since we have been at home, changes have continued but been gradual. We can't get him to say hello, but he did actually start to mumble and make mumbling noises, as if he wanted to say something. Or as if in fact he was saying something, and at times I'd felt he actually thought he had said something to me. He is continent, but that's only because I toilet him regularly. He wears pads, but they very rarely get wet. It's become increasingly difficult to get him out of the chair, but easier to sit him down as he is not so frightened when you are actually sitting him back down again. His jerkiness in the last week or so has increased a lot and I think that has been keeping him awake. The GP has actually increased his Valium, and now he is sleeping all through the night. He seems much calmer and not nearly as jerky during the day.

He is beginning now to have difficulty swallowing his food and he pouches food all the time. Another thing that I've noticed him do is this. He will just open and close his mouth without actually chewing or moving the food around in his mouth. He just does the action of opening and closing, and he has started to dribble quite a lot. I would say that, since he has come out of hospital, his weight has probably stayed about the same: he hasn't lost any weight. I do feel now that sometimes he is having visual disturbances, judging by the way he is squinting his eyes, and the other thing I think is that he is actually having hallucinations, that he is seeing things. He just looks at an empty space and then he will laugh and nod and then look at me, as if to say: "Look at that".

Harash: Yes, I noticed that today.

The other morning when I got up and said: "Hello" to him, he didn't recognise me straight away. It was only when I stop talking to him that he'll recognise me. When I go and give him a kiss, he obviously knows that I'm more friendly. The other morning, he was flinging his arms up in the air, as though trying to warn me off. He looked very disturbed, he was frowning and quite angry, and I felt that he was seeing something that obviously wasn't there. He looked frightened. It was more his trying to fight something off than moving away from it or trying to get away from it. At least, that's how it looked to me. But, after I had talked to him and tried to calm him down and was stroking his arms, he did calm down. Afterwards, he would laugh with me, as if nothing has happened.

The other night, he was sitting in the chair next to me and, all of a sudden, he started moving forward and looking behind, as if he was trying to get away from something. He looked very worried, very frightened, but, once again gain, after talking to him for some time, he did settle down, and he was okay.

Harash: You have cats. Did he ever get frightened of them?

Carol: He doesn't get frightened so much as startled when they jump on him. It's when they jump onto his lap that he gets startled. Now, he doesn't pay the cats as much attention as he did. Whilst he was in hospital, I took the cats into see him. He had one cat sat on his lap for a couple of hours and he was stroking him and holding him. He did that when we first came home as well, but he doesn't pay them much attention at all now.

His perception of space, I think, has altered, because if he is going to step up or down something he takes a bigger step than necessary, and when he is moving around things he takes a wider berth of things than need be.

One thing that I have noticed is that he still responds more to children and if there are children around it makes him very happy. He always has been happy with children but now he tends to overreact with them. If they're running or jumping or getting down from something, he thinks they are falling and he tries to warn them. You've probably noticed a lot of these things today when you've been with Keith.

Harash: Yes, I have. Tell me, the result of the EEG in March was negative. Did they repeat this test and, if they did, what did they find?

Carol: When he was admitted into hospital, he first had an EEG about 7th March, and they repeated it about the 29th March. They said they had noticed considerable change on the EEG, but they didn't explain to me what the changes were. By this time, Keith's condition had deteriorated so much that, maybe they didn't need to tell me, because I could see for myself the changes that were there.

We have always eaten a lot of convenience food because we both work full time. Mind you, if it was ready-made pies for Keith it would have to be chicken. He wouldn't eat meat pies but he might have something like a ready made lasagne. He would eat steak, steak and kidney pie if we went out for a pub meal. Occasionally, we would have beefburgers or steak burgers. We used to have quite a few barbecues in the summer, and we would eat beefburgers then. He would be the one to do the barbecue. To the best of my knowledge, we had not eaten what would contain brain or spinal cord.

Harash: Was there anything unusual in what he ate? You were talking about kebabs.

Yes, that's right, he used to enjoy kebabs, until probably two or three years ago, he might have once a week. Occasionally, he might have made a Chili, using mince. He only had liver twice and that was when I had to persuade him to try it.

Harash: What about his teeth?

He's had fillings, quite a few. In the last few years he has had some fillings done and, in fact, he had great difficulty with one of them. It kept falling out and he had to keep going back to have it redone. He used to get ulcers in his mouth from time to time and little lesions right inside his mouth. He had an abscess many years ago, about twenty years ago, and went to hospital to have it removed. I think the dentist advised him going to the hospital. He said it was too big for him to do. I always thought he felt he had a gastric ulcer or something like that. But then in recent years, in the last three years, I would say that it got worse. He also had Eczema, a dry eczema that he used to get on his wrists. It used to be very bad when he worked with oil and it was worse in the winter and it used to bleed a lot and would get very dried and cracked and he'd get lesions. He bit his nails all the time, used to bite them right down to the quick. You know, he hardly had any nails.

Harash: Now, two more important questions. First of all, you have already told me that you were both blood donors.

Carol: Well, we were both blood donors. I looked at his book actually, because you asked about it, and there's two entries, one for February 1995. That was stamped. The other for May 1995. Now I know for sure that he didn't give blood in May 1995 but they gave him his "25 units certificate", his silver booklet, because he had turned up to give blood but they wouldn't take it because he told them about taking tablets.

The last time he gave blood would have been six months before that. He was a regular blood donor until then. He used to give every six months without fail and then, in the last two years, from about 1993, they asked him to give three times a year.

Harash: Now the second question is this. I've seen the cat sitting on Keith's bed and Keith playing with it. Has he ever been scratched by cats?

Carol: Oh yes. Keith was always the person to be the fondest of the two cats. We have had the cats for about eight years, and, when they were kittens, Keith used to play with them a lot, not so much as they've got older because they are not quite so playful and he has often been scratched by them on his legs and hands.

Harash: Thanks very much for telling me your side of the story.

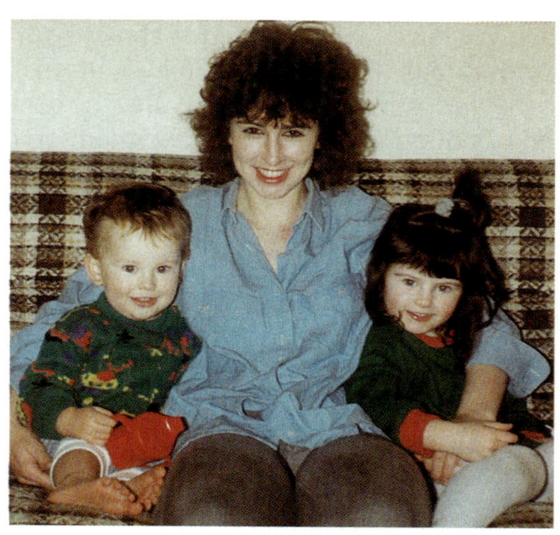

Janice Stuart

Janice Stuart, of Glasgow, Scotland, was a healthy mother of two until CJD struck. The former waitress died, aged 34, in September 1996 after being ill for 11 months. Her fiance described her as "a lovely, wonderful, bubbly girl". She had divorced some years previously. For most of her illness, doctors and psychiatrists treated her for depression.She would fall while walking and had great difficulty balancing herself, typical symptoms of Narang disease. Family suspected she was suffering from mad cow disease and doubted medical diagnosis. They demanded Janice be tested for CJD. Results sent from America the day after she died, confirmed that she was suffering from CJD. She left two children, 7 and 9. Janice's mother, Mrs Stuart and her fiance, Charles Lennon, described seeing Janice's life being taken over by CJD.

Mrs Stuart: My husband and I first noticed a difference in Janice's behaviour back in October 1995. She was never nasty, but she would be snippy. She had got a new house, and I put it down to anxiety, thinking she couldn't cope. But, in fact, she was just a different person, and she seemed withdrawn. If I said: "Janice, what's wrong?" she would say: "I don't know what's wrong".

We noticed a difference in her even before she moved in

October. She seemed to be frightened. She didn't want the children to go out. It was just completely out of character, everything was topsy turvey. That wasn't Janice at all. This wasn't our daughter, the way she was carrying on.

My daughter was a very capable girl, a hard worker and extremely clean. When she got the house, it needed decorating. There was a piece of wallpaper hanging down from the ceiling in her bedroom, and she did nothing about it and that was unlike her. My husband and I thought it really strange, because she was such a particular person. That was really, for me, the first inkling that there was something far wrong with Janice. She caught the flu in the run up to Christmas and got absolutely exhausted.

She used to dress really well, put on her make-up, get her hair done. That changed as well. She would rather just pull on a jersey and trousers.

Everything changed that October. If her dad went over to her house, she would open the door a chink and would just ask him, "What is it?" instead of just opening the door and saying, "Dad, come on in."

It was really weird. Because she wanted to be an independent person in her new house, I didn't go over much. She was only just across the road. When I did go over, I would sit for half an hour and I would think that she would have something she wanted to do, so I would stand up to go away, but she'd just didn't want you to go away. She'd say: "Thank you for your visit, Mum," and get very angry at me for going away. I thought that was ridiculous. I thought she would want to be independent of me, but she wanted me there. She would call me over by phone and say: "Mum, would you come over a minute." I would go over, and I would say: "What is it, Janice?" and she would burst out crying and she would say: "I don't know." She didn't know what was wrong. She knew there was something wrong, but she couldn't say what it was. I thought it was anxiety, not being able to cope. Then I apologised and said: "I am sorry Janice."

It just went on from there, this lack of energy. She was absolutely exhausted every day. That's when I started to do things for her, such as washing and ironing, which, in the past, she would have done. I did it to help, because I could see that she was easily exhausted which seemed unreal.

She had a job during the day, so any work she had to do in her own home had to be done at night, but she was too tired to do anything. That was the problem, her exhaustion was a terrible thing.

I think it was about February, when we thought she had not recovered from the flu, which had made Janice low. I don't think she had ever had flu before in her life. I am not so sure whether it was just flu or something else. In the past, if she had a bad cold, no matter how ill she was, she would drag herself out to work. But she was actually in bed, and that was very unusual for Janice. The weeks were going on, but Janice wasn't getting any better. Her exhaustion continued.

She would ask me if I wanted a cup of coffee, and I would go and make it. She was too tired. It was terrible, she was just too tired. Anything in the house that needed doing, she was just too exhausted to do. She couldn't do anything. I would make her coffee, too. She never finished it: she'd take a few sips and put it down, and in the end I would have to pour it down the sink.

Early on that year, I noticed her staggering as if she was drunk, staggering to one side. She always wanted me to go shopping with her. She was obviously frightened to go on the bus on her own. She was definitely staggering and she would take hold of my arm to steady herself.

She had also been suffering hyperventilation. We knew nothing about that at first. It first happened when Charles met Janice over two years ago. We'd never experienced anything like that before. Her face turned grey, she had this terrible pain, she was gasping for breath. I put it down to the birth pill because we knew there was mood swings with this particular pill, and I said to Janice at the time, "I think you should stop taking that pill." She was blaming the pill for giving her this pain, but the pill obviously had nothing to do with it. It's only in retrospect that you realise. We just jumped to the wrong conclusion, we thought it was the pill and it wasn't.

Janice had been receiving psychiatric treatment for some time as an out-patient. In June 1996, she was admitted to the local hospital where the medical experts believed she had depression. I asked the doctor outright about CJD. I suspected it was CJD.

That was before my husband died in May. There had been a programme about BSE and it described the symptoms: loss of memory, falling about, all of that. John and I looked at one another, and he said to me: ‘That’s Janice’. I said: ‘I know, that is exactly Janice.’ I have had that in my head for a long long time.

We were told: “No.” When Janice was admitted on June 11th to the hospital, I asked the doctor the same question but he also said: “No,” They were quite definite about it.

I told them what I’d seen on the television: I told them about my husband and I talking about it, but they dismissed it completely out of hand. They obviously didn’t think it was CJD. They just said that Janice’s symptoms were bizarre. That was the word they used to me, ‘bizarre’. I am sure that some definitely did have their suspicions.

We didn’t know for certain what Janice had at that time. It was the fact that she was going to be starved that really upset me: she wasn’t eating. The weight was falling off her and, although the thought of CJD was in my head, I was still being told that she had depression.

She was transferred to the Southern General hospital, and, two or three days later, they diagnosed it as ‘dementia’. I’ll never forget it as long as I live. It was such a shock. I got some courage and asked: “Is it hospital policy to call it one thing, when it’s another. Is it going to be a cover-up here, or is the public going to be told.” But the chap never answered me.

She was getting bruises because she was falling all over the place. She couldn’t walk straight. She would walk with her head forward. Her toes were turned in, her toes were curled under her foot; she wasn’t walking properly. By June, when she was seeing a psychiatrist, she could hardly walk. Either I, or a nurse, had to take her to the toilet and she was falling. We thought it was bizarre. The head nurse was absolutely dumb-founded had never experienced anything like it and was very upset. The whole staff were very upset about Janice, because they couldn’t help her. They were giving her pills, but it was doing her no good. She was getting worse, and her memory had gone by this time. She knew us, but she didn’t remember that her dad was dead. He died in May, and she didn’t even remember he was dead.

She wouldn't remember what had happened two minutes ago She remembered the children. She knew them right up until about a month before she died. She would not know their date of birth. She knew their faces, she knew they were her children.

By June, she had stopped feeding herself. She wasn't eating; she was picking at her food. Charles, her fiance, would try to hide this from me because he'd always try and make me feel good. "She'd a good dinner today," he'd say. But I knew differently.

She had her dinner put down in front of her, and she'd pick up the fork and have a bit of this and a bit of that, but she never ever finished her dinner. If it was fish, she would have a little bit, but she could hardly hold the fork by this time. She started having difficulty holding a fork in April, and probably before that. The nurses would feed her, or, at least try to feed her.

She would find drinking a problem too. I asked whether they were going to wait until Janice's kidneys packed up before they put her on a drip. The doctor just smiled; he knew I was upset. They took a blood test every few days because they knew she was becoming dehydrated, but she was not quite dehydrated. This was because, when I went up to the hospital, she would take a drink from me or from Charles, but she would not allow the nurses near her. I was up every day, so she got a small drink every day and even if it was only half a glass, that kept her above the level of being dehydrated, and Charles did the same. We spent hours just asking her to take a sip. That was a very bad time.

A doctor came from the CJD unit in Edinburgh. We were with him for four hours, going into the background of Janice's life from when she was a young girl. At the end of it all, he said to me: "Mrs Stuart, I am 99.9 per cent sure, and I am very sorry to tell you, that your daughter has got CJD." But he also mentioned something which I still want an answer to and want to know more about.. That could be due, he told us, to a faulty gene.

***Janice's fiance, Charles Lennon, who had been with her for more than two years, tried to help her cope with CJD. He describes his experiences of her suffering*.**

Charles: Janice had the flu in October 1995. I didn't think she really recovered from it because afterwards she seemed to get very funny mood swings. We went to the doctor and they told us it was depression. Then she was back at work as a waitress in the country house hotel. Before that, she had been a very strong girl, she wouldn't let anything worry her, she'd carry on. Very strong, unbelievably strong.

Her mood swings were gradually getting worse and worse, and she was getting tired, very tired, exhausted, couldn't be bothered. Then, in January or February, her memory started to go slightly and she was forgetting things. When she was doing her waitressing job, she would be asked for three coffees, and she'd come back and say: 'What was that?' She'd forgotten. And she was getting more and more tired, and her mood swings more and more terrible. They were getting worse.

She didn't know what was wrong with her. She just kept getting tired and wanted to sleep. It was devastating watching her. She got signed off work by the doctor in January or February. Then, two nurses came out and she was prescribed drugs. They thought it was depression. She saw a psychiatrist every fortnight. Then, they upped the dose, but it wasn't doing her any good at all. She was gradually getting worse and worse.

She started to lose her feet: she was getting unsteady on her feet. When she was at home, she would try to wash dishes, and would drop plates. She dropped things all the time. In January she was dropping stuff and into February she was doing that all the time, dropping things and breaking them. They upped her drug dosage and then she came to the cottage here with me in March and I looked after her. She was becoming very unsteady and she was getting hallucinations, thinking she wasn't in a certain place, she was somewhere else and going back, going back to where she was a long time ago. All these things were coming back to her and she was frightened.

When they decided in June that she was to go in to the Ridley Hospital - that's a psychiatric hospital you understand - they were treating her for depression. They were giving her temazepam and they kept putting them into her but she was getting worse. She was walking backwards and walking forwards and really trotting on. Then she got shifted down to another ward, where they could keep a closer eye on her. She was falling over and getting bruised to bits. She was a terrible mess of bruises. They couldn't look after her there, obviously not, and she was getting the jerky movements by that time.

I put pressure on them. I wanted scans taken. She was lying on the bed and she wasn't eating. She was going off her food very, very quickly and not eating. I was up giving her drinks, and I went up one day and created hell. I said to two male nurses at the hospital, "I'm not happy about this." A friend who was with me said: "Charles is asking you now, is she dying?" and they said: "No, it's not life threatening." That's what they said to us.

They did a brain scan. And then, they took her in and gave her another scan because we pressured them - my mother and I pressured them - and then we got an EEG done. This showed there were irregularities in the brain function. They were at last beginning to make some progress after what had been a diabolical state. They were giving her drugs to try and calm her down, but she wouldn't have anyone near her; she'd push and punch at anything.

A month or two later, after she had been taken into the Southern General, she was given another test, a lumbar puncture test in addition to all the different other tests, to eliminate the possibility of all know neurological diseases. She also became incontinent. They were keeping her there and were giving her all the tests, until finally, we were told by the doctor - who pulled us in a corner and told us - that she had got CJD.

They had done another two or three EEGs before we were told it was CJD. Then they told us. I still couldn't believe it, and I fought on and on, and tried to eradicate it from my brain altogether. I was only looking for light at the end of the tunnel to see her get better, but she only got worse and worse.

The doctor told me there were no chances for her. I couldn't believe it. I was still hoping until the day before she died. But that is exactly what happened. It was devastating, terrible.

What if she'd been in a car crash a year ago? She was a healthy young woman who liked the idea of donating organs. I would have said to them, "Take everything that you can of Janice's, so that somebody else can live." What about all these organs had they been transplanted into somebody else's body? Would they have carried the infection?

Harash: What about her teeth?

She had one filling. She had very bad tonsillitis as a young girl and her skin used to break out like eczema.

You asked what she used to eat and what food she enjoyed. Well, it was burgers, Janice just loved a beefburger or a cheeseburger. Not in the house. I didn't make them but I know she often bought them. Spaghetti Bolognese and mince was another of her favourites but it was always the best meat she bought. We would go to the open market at weekends. I always bought mince and never gave it a second thought. We loved pate and steak while she would have burgers in for the children.

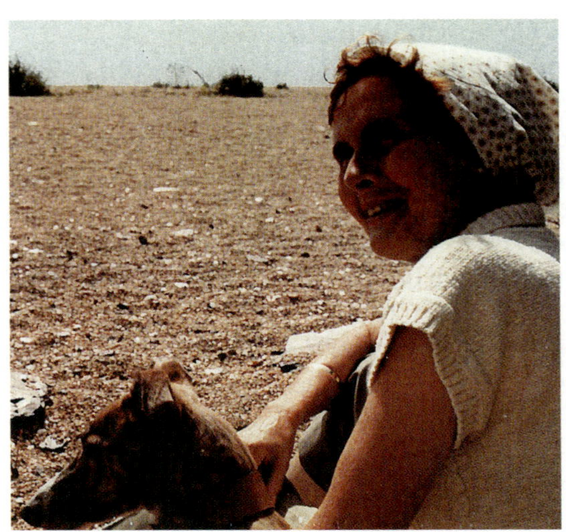

Iris Harris

Iris Harris age 66 died suffering from CJD in Kendal March 1994. Her husband Percy Harris who cared and looked after her during her 6 months illness. He describes the frustrations he had to suffer while she was being investigated while having typical Narang disease symptoms depression, falling over and having difficulty walking. Percy because he did not know what CJD was, the hospital doctor explains that this was his second case and he was explained that his wife was suffering from similar disease as mad cow disease. Percy talks to Harash Narang of his frustrations during the course of diagnosis and he had to live now with the scar and fear.

We were married 25 years and all that time she was in perfect health and had never had any operation. The trouble all began about the beginning of September, 1993. Iris my wife had a dose of flu but had got over that. She was in the best of health, a lot healthier than me and very bright with a fantastic memory. She had been a private secretary most of her working life, and could speak a number of foreign languages.

It was a few weeks after she had got over the flu and was perfectly O.K. A few days later she suddenly said: "Oh, I do feel poorly, I feel depressed, I feel rotten. I have got no energy." She was just getting up and doing the housework and then sitting down and taking more rests than she normally did. It wasn't only the once she said it at about that time, the beginning of September, she said: "I do feel poorly, Am I ill?" I said: "Oh you're all right, you're always being bloody funny." I just laughed it off. In a matter of days, she said to me, "We're not daft are we." We just had a quiet chuckle. She knew there was something wrong but, of course, she'd no idea what the trouble was. She didn't make a big thing about it but I could see she wasn't her old self. You know, I, myself am not young; it was difficult and hard, but I tried to do everything for her.

A week or two after that she started doing the odd silly thing, and I used to look at her and think, "That's odd", and used to say to her "What's wrong with you". Well, I could see there was something the matter, but she never complained about anything herself. Her eye sight began to deteriorate. She said: "I think I'll have to have my glasses changed, they don't seem to be strong enough." But, her sight continued to get worse. She couldn't read at all. That was all within a few weeks of her getting over the flu. When she continued to get worse I had the doctor in to see her. The doctor did not know of her eyesight problem. He didn't ask and I didn't think it was relevant.

Another thing, she had trouble with was her balance, and that must have started about the time of the flu. She would stand with her feet wider apart than normal. She said to me, "I'm dizzy". She became shaky and unsteady on her feet. About two weeks from the start, she was spending more and more time in bed. I said: "You're getting worse, not better." She agreed.

I did not want her trailing down to the surgery in the condition she was in, so I called the doctor in. He came to have a look at her. He said there was nothing wrong with her other than the after-effects of the flu. I told the doctor here that she had lost her sense of balance and couldn't stand and she certainly couldn't walk. I used to have to lift her up, and hold her, and sit her in a chair. Later on, I virtually had to carry her to the bathroom because she wasn't capable of walking on her own. If she wanted to go to the toilet she had to be literally carried.

I said: "No, no there's more to it than that: she was over the flu. She is worse now than when she had the flu." The doctor said: "Well, that's all it is", and away he went. Well, in the following week, she got rapidly worse, she went off her food. I had a hell of a job to get anything into her and at the end of another week she had difficulty swallowing. She just didn't want food, but of course she was still drinking.

At the end of fourth week, I called the doctor again and he was a bit short with me. He came in and looked at me and said: "Well, there's nothing wrong with her. I told you before its just the residue of the flu." I said: "She is getting rapidly worse. There is something seriously wrong." Ridiculous, he said: "Are you trying to tell me my job?"

I said: "Well I think it's time somebody did because there is something sadly wrong with my wife."

He carried on about how many patients he had to look after, and all the rest of it. We had a few words actually and he went. Before he went, I said: "She isn't eating, she's gone off her food." "Oh well" he said: "That's quite normal, but there's no need to worry as long as she drinks plenty." So, I asked "What do you call plenty?" "Three litres a day," he said. I said: "Do you drink three litres a day? She's loosing her energy, she's wasting away already."

"Oh that is just lack of exercise." So away he went.

Well, we struggled on for another week. I was getting really vexed because she was going downhill rapidly. She was starting to do all sorts of silly things. Her memory had gone, her balance had gone, she couldn't walk. By the end of the fifth week, I was literally carrying her to the toilet. Her speech went. She couldn't pronounce some words, she couldn't get her tongue round them. Everything was slowing up for her and she would nod to mean "Yes" but be unable to say it. So I called the doctor again.

The senior partner came. He said: "What's the matter with her, Percy." I told him I didn't know but there was something drastically wrong with her. He gave her a fairly decent examination: he certainly did spend more time than the previous fellow.

After the examination he said to me, "This lass is short of protein and she's short of exercise." I said: "How can she get exercise when she can't even stand." I said: "You talk just as daft as the other doctor did." Well, he was a bit taken aback at that but said: "See what you can do with her over the weekend and, if you aren't happy, give me another ring on Monday."

So, I said to him, “It’s not my job to try and do something with her. You’re the bloody doctor.” Anyway it didn’t make any difference. I mean they didn’t know what the hell they were doing: they didn’t know what to do, and that was the top and bottom of it. I sort of fiddled over the weekend.

Monday, I rang up for the doctor and played merry hell. The doctor did come on Tuesday, but not in the morning, as he was supposed to do, but after I had gone to work leaving a friend, Kath, to watch my wife. She told me about the doctor’s visit after I got home - “Oh, well, just after you’d gone, the doctor came. He just looked at Iris, took one look and said: could he use the telephone. She has to go into hospital tonight”.

So we took her to the hospital at night - and it was a hell of a struggle, first of all in the car, and then up to the ward in a wheel-chair. She was under a really nice bloke. I saw him the following day and we both wanted to speak to each other. He said: “I have got to tell you at the outset that your wife is very ill indeed.” I said: “I know that, I’ve been telling our GP that for three weeks. They kept trying to fob me off with the fact that it was the aftermath of the flu.” He said: “God! To be honest, I don’t know what’s wrong with her. I’ve put her on some drug, that won’t cure anything, but what I propose to do is to send her down for a brain scan to Lancaster. That should show something and, if it doesn’t, we will then do a lumbar puncture. Between one and the other, we’ll get to the bottom of it.”

She went down to Lancaster for a brain scan but it didn’t show anything. The lumbar puncture they did did not show anything either. So he said: “There’s something serious going on.” I asked: “Where do we go from here?” He said: “Well I’m going to send her for another brain scan, but not to Lancaster because they’ve missed things before. I’ll send her down to Preston.” That was on a Friday. They took her down by ambulance and she had this scan and they brought her back that night. Then, they admitted her to Preston Hospital the following day.

In Preston Hospital they twice did a test called EEG. There was a rapid deterioration between the first one and the second one and that was over a period of only a week or ten days. She deteriorated very, very quickly. She had these jerky things which she had not had when she was at home. I went down to see the doctor. He said: "I'm not going to raise your hopes. I don't think there's anything I can do. I don't think there is anything anyone can do." He said: "I want you to spend a bit of time with my assistant. Tell her everything you can remember, right from the beginning and in the right order if you can."

I said: "Yes, OK," because it was fresh in my mind then. I went through it. When I saw him the second time he said: "I have put your wife on a drug but, quite honestly, I don't think it's going to do any good. We've had success with this in other cases, but not with the same sort of problems your wife's got. It's the only thing I can possibly do, but don't hold out any hopes because I don't think there's any thing anyone can do." "I know what the problem is", he said: "and what she's got, but we can't do anything about it." So I said: "Well, what has she got." He said: "It's CJD."

"Well I'd never heard of that before. I had to ask him what it was and why there was no treatment for it. He explained to me that it was similar to "mad cow" disease. Naturally, I had heard of mad cows disease. So I said: "How did you know that."

He told me, "I've only dealt with one case before, and I've only known of three cases in my working life. In this hospital, I'm the only person that's dealt with one." So I said: "In that case, how do you know that my wife's got it."

He said: "You, you clever bugger, you gave me the clue. You told me that she started to do silly things with her right hand. She started to move her wrists and her hands and her fingers in such a funny way, that's right. That's it, they want to get there but its twisting. That's put me onto it. She would get rapidly worse and she'd be bedfast. There was no hope: it was just a matter of ticking over until she dies. It could be three months to eighteen months."

He asked: "If it comes to the point where we have to do something drastic to keep her alive, what do we do?" I said: "Well if there's no hope of recovery and she's getting in the state that she's in now, forget it, forget it, it will do no-one any good."

He said: "It's a situation, we can't encourage the end, but we do delay the end. There isn't any point in this case. There's a doctor from Edinburgh will want to come and talk to you. We'll let you know."

Dr. DeSilva came to see me. He wanted me to complete a lengthy questionnaire and a lot of what he asked seemed irrelevant, although I suppose they've got to get all the facts down.

When he told me that Iris had got CJD, he asked me to keep it quiet. He said: "Don't shout it out, its just between us. Keep it just within the immediate family." So I said: "Why, what's the point of that." He said: "Well, if the press got hold of it, they'll make a hell of a meal of it. You don't want to be hounded by the press do you." I said: "What do I do if people ask me what she's got." "Oh, just tell them she's got a very rare illness, a rare virus" said the doctor.

So I said: "That's all very well, but, surely, I can tell the truth?" He said: "Just think what it would do to our bloody meat trade." I said: "I'm not concerned about the meat trade." He was a hell of a nice bloke, but I didn't agree with that attitude. Thinking of the implications for the meat trade, to hell with the meat trade. He said: "Iris could have had this virus inside her body for years." I said: "How many years." He said: "I don't know —five, ten, fifteen, twenty, even twenty five years."

So I said: "Well, why does it suddenly start up now then." "Oh", he said: "I wish we knew." He said something had triggered it off - possibly shock. I had a slight accident not long before it all started with Iris but that was after her trouble had begun. Admittedly, if she had been fit and well when I had that accident she would have been upset but, by that time, she was a the stage of not really appreciating anything about anything. My accident made no real impression on her: she was past it.

Anyway, the doctor at the Preston Hospital said he'd do what he could to save a lot of hassle and a lot of trouble. They would make her as comfortable as they could and then move her back to Kendal to be nearer for you. I thought he was a great bloke. He was straight and he didn't pull his punches.

She lost, her voice towards the end. Oh Lord, yes. She went rapidly down from the time they diagnosed her in Preston, but she came back to Kendal and she died last March, just over a year ago and since then I've heard of more and more cases.

I think there's a lot more of CJD than people realise and that the authorities are not letting on. They gave me some pamphlet to read in Preston and it said there that obviously this was the human equivalent of BSE and BSE was the cattle equivalent of Scrapie in sheep and they've know about that since 1760, or something like that. Well I've known of scrapie but up here they call it scurvy. But, obviously, you don't connect these things if you are not involved.

Quite honestly, we didn't eat a lot of meat, we ate more poultry than meat. What I can't understand this is, if it comes through what we ate, why did my wife get it and I did not get. That brought it home to me again that there were a lot more cases than the Government were letting on. This literature they gave me to read while I was at Preston said this was a very rare disease and affected only one out of every two million people.

Harash: What was the condition of her teeth?

She'd had two teeth removed many years ago so she had a little plate with two teeth on but all the time I've known her she went to the dentist every six months and she never needed anything doing. Well, going back a few years now, she used to put some antiseptic in her throat. I remember she used to put it on her tongue, fold her tongue back to reach it.

Harash: Would she recognise you when you went to see her and other people, those who went to visit her.

Yes, in the early days, yes, but she was only in Kendal here for about ten days. She was perfectly OK. In fact she was eating a little bit except that she couldn't go to the toilet on her own but she did recognise us. Then she went down to Preston and in a matter of days she didn't even know we were there, never mind recognise us. It was so rapid.

You were asking about what food she ate. We didn't eat a lot of minced up stuff because you could never know what it was. She ate a lot of fish and chicken and, occasionally, ham. She was far more finicky about her food than her mother had been. Iris was brought up in Congleton, Macclesfield and you know what people up there are like for food. Lancashire Hot and Yorkshire Puddings. Her mother would eat anything and everything and I suppose Iris ate the same to begin with. They'd boil bones, sometimes with the head left on, and let them simmer and simmer with vegetables. That didn't appeal to me.

Her father worked in one of the local mills. He died of a heart complaint in 1995 - 56. Her mother and her sister both died not many years ago. Well they were both in their 80s but that's the age when you expect them to suffer a bit.

With the aunt and her mother, not very rapid. I know that it was..... Six months, a year. It was coming for quite some time. Something I would call a normal process of aging. It wasn't any rapid deterioration at all. None of these balancing symptoms and things, just a simple memory loss. Gradual loss of memory. The first time, we thought that she was just being bloody awkward. We went to South Wales and when we got there I had booked her into this local hotel and we drew up with the caravan behind. We still had to go onto the site and she flatly refused to stay. She said: "I'm going home". I said: "How are you going to go home". "I'll go on the train or I'll hitch-hike". We had a hell of a job to get her inside the hotel and we were dreading it. When we went to pick her up the following morning expecting all hell to be let loose. We found her sitting with a whisky in front of her. She said: "Hey, come in, Percy, its smashing here. They'll give you a drink at any time. That was the first instance that we had that something was not quite right.

I think the next time that it really came home to us was, I think, somewhere in Scotland. We were on the site and she said: "I want to go to the toilet, which way is it. It's in that direction Florrie, but she was absolutely lost. She didn't know where the devil she was and of course we both swore at her and said: "Don't be stupid, but it was only later we realised that she just honestly didn't know. We would have had a lot more consideration for her if we had only realised.

Harash: Now tell me, another thing. You've got two pets, you've had them all the time?

We've always had dogs yes. We feed them with tinned meat but mostly it's this, "All in One" we give them, this modern dried food, vegetables and meat. To begin with we used to give them a bone every now and again but unless we knew how fresh they were, we weren't very keen on that.

I do want to mention the Death Certificate they gave for Iris. I asked one of the doctor's, what would be shown on the Certificate and he said: "Well ,its most unlikely that they will put CJD". That was in the hospital and he would have been one of the Consultants. I insisted that CJD be recorded on the death certificate.That brought me another problem as well when I went to register the death because the Registrar in that office said: "What's this CJD? I've never heard of it."

I told her "Well its this mad cows diseases." "Oh my God." she said: "Has the Coroner been informed?" "No", I said: "Oh", she said: "we'll have to ring him." "What the hell for, You've got a death certificate, what more do you want. "Oh, but I'll have to inform him." I said: "I've already been here now an hour and a half waiting." She said: "I don't know how to spell it, I'll have to ring him to find out how to spell it." I said: "The spellings on the death certificate." So anyway I got it eventually, but it was the first time she'd come across it . Whether she finally phoned the Coroner or not I don't know, but she didn't phone him when I was there.

Harash: Did they do a post mortem?

Maybe it would have brought into the public domain. Now this is not the first time that I've heard this story I've heard it a few times that people have been led up the garden path you know, when they didn't say what it should be they led them round and round trying to see whether they would be happy with something else. Like the guy said you know, don't tell anybody. Yes, that's right, keep it quiet. Do you think they're doing it to more patients, or just pretending.

Harash: I don't know. I've got nothing to substantiate but I have a feeling that there is more of this than the public are aware of. Who do you think they are being told by? Doctors would be honest you know.

Our eating habits have changed. Now, we have rice, jacket potatoes, but we still eat pork, lamb and chicken.

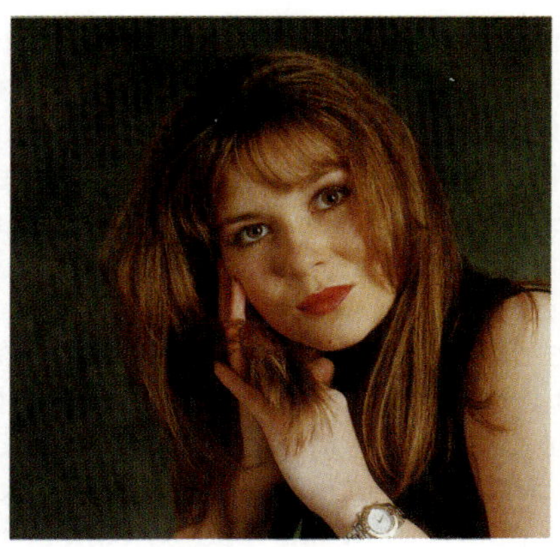

Victoria Lowther

After being ill for about 10 months, Victoria, an out-going girl, died at the age of 19. Her clinical symptoms had been those of Narang disease: depression, balancing difficulties and shaking reminiscent of that seen in BSE cattle. She was treated in the RVI, Newcastle upon Tyne, the same hospital as Peter Hall. After a number of tests, she was first suspected as suffering from ME and, later, from a brain tumour. Eventually, Victoria was diagnosed as suffering from CJD. She had no links with any known source of that disease, such as infected growth hormone and there was no history of the disease in her family. Looking back to the time, Patricia, her mother, recalls the feeling of being left unsupported and on her own, with nobody to help or counsel the family with the difficulties they faced. The family just felt angry and very frustrated. Although, Victoria was clinically diagnosed suffering from CJD, no advice was given on the importance of a post- mortem and, therefore,none was performed. Victoria's death is, therefore, not included in the CJD Surveillance statistics.

Patricia her mother talks to Harash Narang after Victoria died.

Patricia: Victoria Louise Lowther was a nineteen year old girl, full of life, with everything going for her. She had a family who adored her and was a very independent teenager,with a sparkling, bubbly personality. She completed her "A" Level exams, and left school when she was 18 years old to start working as a Customer Liaison Executive for Conway Vauxhall in Carlisle. She loved the work and put everything into it, successfully launching the Vauxhall Vectra in October 1995, for which she received letters of appreciation from the company.

In February 1996, she started being unwell, just complaining about tiredness. I took her backward and forward to the doctor a few times. Different tests were done and the doctor advised Victoria to get a tonic from the health shop. We went through lots of tonic, but that didn't help Victoria at all. The doctor tried all kinds of other tests, but nothing helped. I took her back again to the doctor in March and yet more tests were done. By this time, she was so poorly that she had to cancel her holiday and she started to worry about her job, complaining to me that the girls at work were "getting at her". She said that, from time to time, she could not remember what to do. All I could do as her mother was advise her to write things down. I thought that would help.

Often, I heard her crying in the shower before she went to work, and it was becoming very obvious that she was unhappy with what she was doing. I advised her to change her job in the hope that this would help sort out her work-related problems. At this time, she showed no physical signs of illness. On my advice, she applied for a job with Volvo garage in Carlisle, and succeeded in getting the job. After only a few weeks there, the same problems surfaced again. I found her crying and she was lacking interest in working with her colleagues. It was obvious that something wasn't right, and, though at this stage, she didn't look ill, I took her back to the doctors. Some routine tests were carried out, blood tests and blood pressure levels, and subsequently, Victoria was diagnosed as suffering from M.E. Victoria then left this second job at Volvo as she just felt unable to cope with the pressures of every day life at work.

I noticed that, day by day, Victoria's body was slowing down. She had previously worn the most fashionable clothes and token pride in her appearance. Now, she had to be urged to wash her hair and keep herself clean. She would answer the telephone but then be unable to remember who she had spoken to. Her walking became awkward and we began to think that she had a brain tumour. Her reactions were slow, and I stopped her from driving her car as I felt she was not fully in control of the vehicle. Her mood swings were uncontrollable: she would shout and push me, something that had never happened before. She became quite irritable with her younger brother, Mark and his presence seemed to anger her. Most of her reactions were against him.

I do recall one incident in April, 1996 when Victoria was planning a holiday with her boyfriend, Simon, and she seemed confused about paying for her holiday. She told me that she was short of money. We both were in the Town Centre at the time and Victoria began to cry, saying that she couldn't afford to go on holiday. Then she said: "I am £50 short". I said: "That's only £25 each, so what are you panicking about?" Victoria began shouting and pushed me before running off leaving me standing on me own. This was totally out of character. She and I were very close. She went home and told her father she'd had a "ballistic" with her mum and then went straight to her boyfriend's house. Normally, Victoria would have phoned to apologise, but this time she did not bother. Next day, she walked into the house as if nothing had happened.

At this time my husband, Stanley, Victoria's father and I began to wonder if she was taking drugs, despite having no reason to suspect it. There were a couple of times when Victoria had arranged to meet her friend Sarah in town but she forgot and Sarah had to phone up looking for her. Her behaviour was abnormal, and, naturally, we began to think that something was very seriously wrong with her.

We were thinking about going away for a holiday and I telephoned our local GP to ask what he thought about the idea. He said that it would do Victoria good to get away, so, in July 1996, Stanley and I with Victoria and Mark all went to Majorca for 2 weeks. During that holiday, Victoria completely changed from being independent and outgoing to dependent and lethargic. She became clingy and wanted to sleep with me. She now even needed help getting out of chairs and support to steady her when she was walking. Although she had loved swimming, she made no attempt to get into the pool, even though given every encouragement to do so.

I began doing everything for Victoria, from running her bath to deciding what she was going to wear. It was just as though she had gone back to her childhood. She could still eat with a knife and fork, but her conversation tailed off and she began fidgeting. She could not lie still and her legs moved constantly and erratically when she was in bed. When she walked, she bumped into me, and at the end of the two weeks holiday, she needed to be supported on both sides to walk.

When we arrived home in August 1996, Victoria was taken to see an M.E. specialist in Newcastle. He spent a long time examining her and watching her movements. He even video-taped her walking. He asked lots of questions, most of which I had to answer and was told not to. He wanted to hear how Victoria could respond. At the end of the examination, the specialist told us that Victoria was not suffering from M.E. and that, in his opinion, she was suffering from a disease called "St Vitus Dance". This is an old fashioned illness, but Victoria had the appropriate symptoms. Once back home in Carlisle, I contacted her GP and arranged for Victoria to go and see him, and discuss what the specialist had said. As Victoria walked into the surgery, I recall the look on the doctors face. His face visibly changed. It was then we realised that there was more to it than the specialist had diagnosed and told us. After Victoria's death, the GP told me that it was then, in his surgery, that he suspected for the first time one or other of several illnesses. One of these was CJD. The next day he telephoned to tell me he had not slept all night worrying about Victoria and that he was trying to get her into hospital for more tests. This devastated me and Stan, because, although we suspected something was seriously wrong, it was then that the reality of the situation suddenly hit us. That morning, Victoria was taken to the Cumberland Infirmary where, the next day, a consultant from Newcastle, a neurologist, was taking a clinic. He examined Victoria and afterwards wanted her to go to Newcastle immediately. Unfortunately, as there was no ambulance then available, Victoria was only taken to the Royal Victoria Infirmary Newcastle the following morning. Various tests were carried out and many illnesses were ruled out, including AIDs and Parkinson's Disease. They also confirmed that she was not pregnant. Scans of Victoria's brain activity were monitored but showed nothing wrong.

On September 6th 1996 a further brain scan was done when grey areas were discovered on the brain. I asked the consultant about this and was told that it was indeed serious and that further investigation was needed. We asked if it was a tumour, and he said: “No”. We became frantic as more and more tests were carried out. I asked that consultant whether it could be CJD and he said that that could not be ruled out and he was going to make it his next test. For this, a man came from the CJD unit in Edinburgh to talk to us and he took spinal fluid from Victoria which was sent to America for testing. The man from the unit spent about 2 hours with us asking lots of questions, in particular about the food Victoria ate. We felt he knew she was suffering from CJD, and asked him how long from the onset of the illness to the end. He said we could expect it to be about a year. My husband and I both felt he was a very cold uncaring character.

When we returned to the hospital 10 days later, Dr Bates told us the good news that the test for CJD was negative, but 2 days later, we were told that it had, in fact, proved positive. The American test is not a sophisticated one and, while it is reckoned to detect CJD in most cases, it is not 100% reliable and foolproof.

By this time, Victoria’s illness was well developed. Her balance was completely gone and she was in a wheelchair. Her conversation was limited to only the occasional word. The RVI in Newcastle could do little for her and, to be closer to home, it was decided that Victoria should be transferred back to the Cumberland Infirmary. Once again, there was no ambulance available and this infuriated us and we decided that, rather than going back to the Carlisle Hospital we would take her home and nurse her ourselves. That we did and the District nurses called in to help bath her in the mornings. Our GP and these nursing staff were very kind and helpful and we very much appreciate the help they gave us. We visited the Hospice to discuss respite care for Victoria and used it a few times.

The saddest thing was Victoria lost all her personality and was so terribly helpless, unable to recognise people, slipping backwards to become more like a little girl again and having to have every thing done for her. She had to be bathed, fed and changed, just like a baby. Happily, she had no pain with this illness and didn't suffer. Frankly,we don't believe she was even aware of what was happening to her and, in her case, the illness in this case ended quickly.

We were lucky. We are reasonably comfortably off and had been able to give her a private education which she enjoyed in a school where she ended up as deputy head girl. Her future should have been wonderful. Instead, we are left heartbroken and wondering what there is to look forward to and how to go on. In her short lifetime, Victoria touched a lot of people and we never saw so many men cry as on the day of her funeral. It just doesn't make sense and, without that, you cannot come to terms with it.

Victoria died on November 19th 1996 very peacefully, in her sleep. That was a blessing. On her gravestone her parents have written "IF ONLY WE HAD BEEN GIVEN ONE WISH"

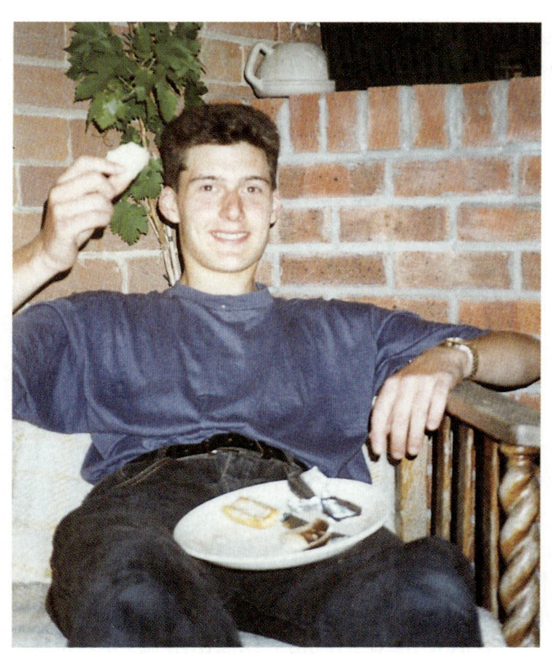

Stephen Churchill

At the age of 19, Stephen Churchill died from the new variant of CJD in May 1995. The Lancet medical journal published his case in October 1995 and this immediately rang alarm bells. Sporadic CJD usually strikes people far older, and Stephen had no links with known sources of the disease, such as infected growth hormone. Stephen had typical symptoms of Narang disease and was being looked after by the same consultant as Donald who had growth hormone treatment with similar symptoms as Stephen and was diagnosed CJD without difficulty. His father, David, said at the time: "The Government keeps saying that there is no evidence of a link with BSE, but we say there is No evidence of no link." Just five months later the link with BSE was admitted by Government scientists and ministers to be highly probable. Stephen sister, Helen, said: "I was just sat at home having my lunch after I had been to college one day, and it took a while for me to realise, but there was actually somebody on television telling me that my brother had died because of something he'd eaten. And I just felt so angry and very frustrated, and it was just completely out of the blue. Nobody had warned us that anything was going to be said: and there was an MP stood there saying that Steve had died from beef." David and Dot, Stephen's mother, of Devizes in Wiltshire, talk to me while Stephen was still alive. They talked about what led up to Stephen's early death, and because of great doubts as to what was going on asked me to be present at their son's post-mortem. A day after Stephen post-mortem, I confirmed to his parents that Stephen's death was due to CJD.

Harash: Tell me the way you think when it started. What changes did you see? Go back as far as you can accurately remember, it doesn't really matter where you start. It may be at times very distressing. I hope you understand that.

Dot: We've been through it so many times that, hopefully, we can recount it reasonably well, right from the start of our noticing that something was going wrong. After all, Stephen had always been a pretty healthy kid. He had very little time off school, only the odd cough and cold. The only operations he had was when he was eight years old when he had all his toes straightened. To begin with, we thought Stephen was suffering from depression. That was the opinion of his teachers and the doctor. We then thought quite carefully about what had gone before and at various stages discussed with doctors and many times sought second and third opinion. It is just four days ago that we heard how to contact you. Well we thought we would contact you and see if what we had been told over the last six months was true. You might be able to tell us more about CJD. We have a lot of questions we'll want to ask you.

Dave: In November 1993, about a year before his first symptoms appeared, Stephen went to RAF Cranwell for a sixth-form scholarship. He always wanted to join the Royal Air Force and was already an air cadet. He went through four days of testing and was passed as flying-fit and had flying aptitudes. However, his upper leg was too long to allow him to fit into a Hawk aircraft without taking his lower leg off if he ejected. They would not allow him to go forward as a pilot or navigator. They suggested that he thought about trades other than joining the RAF and he did not get a six-months scholarship.

Around February, he was invited to go to RAF Boulmer,

Northumberland to have a look at fighter control because they felt he was suitable for a high-pressure, high-reaction job. He spent two nights up there in the officers' mess and thoroughly enjoyed it. He thought fighter control might be for him and they offered him a pilot navigation course to start at Easter 1994.

All the time that was going on, from the period of October 1993, my father was dying of liver cancer in the North East and we were spending a lot of time commuting up there and back, and eventually finding him a nursing home to end his days. This meant that we were away a lot, leaving Stephen to get on with his 'A' level studies.

From Easter he went to RAF Benson, and he had a wonderful time. He came out with a credit, spent two weeks flying with the RAF. He spent his eighteenth birthday there, and had a superb birthday there. He went away for a week for a geography field trip, they went to study the Whitby area and he enjoyed that. Also during the Easter period, he went to his annual camp with the air cadets on Salisbury Plain, and again he thoroughly enjoyed that. He came back absolutely shattered.

My father died on the May 1st after a period of illness but Stephen did not seem too badly affected by it, he did come up for the funeral. He was okay, he was emotional about the funeral cremation service, but not unduly so. He did not seem too deeply affected by it.

He did not do very well in his lower-sixth exams in May, and he had to re-sit one subject at the end of the summer holidays. He went to Salamanca on a Spanish language course for two weeks in August while we went to Sweden on our summer holiday. He contracted salmonella poisoning while there. Stephen came back from Spain on August 19th.

The following Friday evening, August 26th, Stephen went out with a friend in Dot's car, a Fiesta. He was driving along a long straight stretch of a country road and collided with an army four-tonner when he crossed the middle line and suffered minor facial injuries and quite severe shock. They gave him various X-rays and treated him for a head injury and discharged him two or three hours later,with a few stitches.

That crash affected him quite deeply. He felt he had let us

down. It was a very serious accident and he should never have got out of that car without serious injury. When he saw the car the next day, he realised how lucky he had been and was deeply shocked. Soon after that, he went back during the school holiday to re-sit his exam and did not do very well in them. In addition, he did not do the geography project he was supposed to have done over the summer.

He went back to school at the beginning of term, mid-September, and from then his school-work concerned us. He was told to report daily what work he had done and put under close supervision. We were called in for a round-table meeting and Steve said: "Look, I'm not coping with the work, I can't cope with course work." The school was very good with him, and said: "We'll forget course work. We'll change the syllabus, you can do something that does not have exams at the end." However, his results did not improve at all. At another round-table meeting, the school said: "We will get you notes from other students to build up your file, so you have the information you need." But still Steve was not doing well.

He was down in general terms: I would not use the word depressed, but down. He said he had no friends at school, he was quite distraught and on October 18th, we found this letter, which basically said: "I'm a failure. I can't go on. I've let you down, and I am going to leave school." The school rang the next day to say that Steve was showing signs of depression. We had another round-table discussion with the various heads and agreed that Steve had a problem and that we should consider psychotherapy to help him. We were told that it was not unusual in the 'A' level year for this sort of thing to happen. He fitted the model of an 'A' level student under stress. So Steve went, by himself, to a session with a psychotherapist in Bath.

Steve also saw his GP who knew him but she was quite dismissive and gave him the 'pull yourself together and get on with your work' routine. She told Dot: "He's a lad who's never had to work. He went through his GCSE's very easily, and he has to realise there's hard work ahead of him." He pretended to do school-work over half-term, but it was very half-hearted. The next day, we took him to the psychotherapist's. We offered him the choice of one of us going with him, and he said: "No." He came out of there a bit brighter, it seemed.

I used to get up with him, give him his breakfast and get him on the road. He had a fairly early start to catch a coach to Bath. They were our little bits of time together, and we used to chat about whatever came to mind - school, and so on. By this period, he was withdrawn and not communicating, so we just got on with the routine of getting him off to school. All of the warning signs were probably there, but, obviously, I did not understand. The following Friday morning he went out as usual. At 3 o'clock in the afternoon, Dot had a phone call from the school.

Dot: They were waiting for us at the school because Stephen had seen the head teacher that morning and told him he was leaving. He said he had discussed it with us, that we were going in to sign papers, then he was finished. We did not go in, because we knew nothing about it. We dashed into the school, and I said: "Well, where is he?" and they said: "He's gone." We thought he had run off. In fact, he was just sitting in the school library in a kind of daze. He just sat there. He saw us, he did not move. He had an empty expression in his eyes. We again had a brief meeting, and we said: "We'll take him out of school on sick leave, see if we can straighten him out, and see if we can find out what's happening. We may have to take a long break, have a review perhaps after Christmas", but that didn't matter. Steve's welfare was what mattered. We brought him home, and we had a very tearful hour or two discussing his failures, as he saw it, his ability to cope and his attitude to various things.

David: That evening, I did something quite out of character for me, I put my arm around his shoulder - this was obviously quite a landmark day - and said: "We'll just go down the pub and have a couple of drinks, and talk about it." I took him down to the local pub, which is very close by, and he got quite drunk on one-and-a-half pints of larger. At least, it appeared that he was quite drunk on the lager - talking incoherently, nonsensically, and staggering. So we came home.

Harash: This staggering .... Do you mean like a walking off balance. Had you noticed any staggering of any sort before that day or any sign that he was having difficulty making straight towards where he wanted?

Dot: Yes, and I would say that probably started around that

date. The only time that I can think of when Steve staggered before that was on October 1st when we had our 25th wedding anniversary. We had a party and Stephen was letting off some fireworks. He sort of staggered between the fireworks. We thought he had had too much to drink, which he might well have done.

Harash: Let me ask you another question while we're talking about it. Did you see any sort of shakes at the breakfast table in his hand, anything to suggest they were not quite as steady as they should be, trying to put sugar in his tea and the sugar spilling as much on the table or on the saucer as went into his cup?

Dot: No, we hadn't seen that but what we had noticed since the summer he was forever saying, "Pardon." He would often drop it into whatever he was saying, nearly every sentence. It was like a nervous tick.

Dave: On the Thursday, he went to his air cadets and was very aggressive with one of his colleagues. He came in late that night, and I accused him of being drunk, and he said: "No, I didn't even stop on the way home for a drink, we stopped for some chips and that's all. I've had nothing to drink." He said he had not drunk, and I tended to believe him. I only thought he was drunk because he was staggering and slurring his speech. He was slurring in the sense that his tongue was twisting. On the Friday evening, he was partly incoherent, and partly nonsensical and irrational, but he got up on the Saturday morning as normal to go to his Saturday job at a shop in Devizes. He loved the job. He said he had heard that there was a full-time job at the shop, and he was going to go down to see if he could get an interview. We said to him, "Forget about school if you're not happy. We are not going to push you. If you want to get a job, go and do it, whatever's best for you." In fact I watched him walk out of the house and he walked perfectly ordinarily. He came back within about an hour and said he had got an interview for the job. A bit later, he said he was going out that night because he had a bar-job at the pub down the road. He had been to the estate agents who sold our house to us, but they did not have jobs. He said he had been to the police station for an application form for working on a helicopter unit working with the police.

I went to pick my daughter up from the railway station, and when we came back he said: "I'm going out because I'm going to the jewellers."

"Which jewellers?" I asked.

He described the place, but it did not exist, and then we realised something definitely was wrong. He was very, very tired sitting in the chair, and I said: "Why don't you go and have a sleep?" He did not want to, he said: because he was having nightmares. He had had nightmares over the previous few weeks. He was having great difficulty sleeping.

That was it. We just did not know what was going on.

We called our GP out and I had a chat with our doctor. We said we just didn't know what's going on and the first thing the GP wanted to know was had Steve been taking drugs. He didn't mix with anybody with drugs and he never had the money for them. The GP said that parents are the last to know. The doctor had a long chat with Steve, and decided it was depression and gave him tablets to take for about a fortnight. He went back to see the doctor, who upped those to a stronger dose because they were not having any effect.

The psychotherapist at this stage thought it was well out of his league and said Steve should see the psychiatrist at the local mental hospital. Steve by then had got a bit disorientated. If you put a cup down, and said to Stephen to drink his tea, he would cup his hands, but holding no actual cup, and make as though drinking. The psychotherapist said Steve was hallucinating and was disorientated in place and time. He was staggering. He was sleeping an awful lot of the day - up to fifteen hours a day. He would have night-time sleep and a long afternoon sleep. He would watch the television and become enthralled with it, and become frightened by it - absolutely terrified. If there was a threatening situation, he would feel as if he himself was really in it. This happened with simple situations. For example, while watching the programme *Black Beauty*, a child went into a hay-loft and Steve would be anxious that there might be somebody up there. He was absolutely petrified. If somebody was going to be knifed, Steve actually recoiled.

The psychiatrist first gave Steve intelligence-type tests, asking questions such as: when was World War Two? He could answer this kind of question, but he could not tell you what the month was, or what his date of birth was. He could answer historical questions and subjects he had learned from school, such as mental arithmetic. But he could not remember things which had happened on that day. The doctor eventually changed Steve's drugs, which did not help him.

Christmas was drawing near. As Dave and I were on holiday, and as both of us were at home, we decided we would keep Stephen at home over Christmas. The psychiatrist said that there was a bed for him in the hospital but we said: "No." We kept him at home, but he did not join in the Christmas festivities. I do not think he even saw the Christmas tree in the corner. He just had lots of sleep.

Dave: Steve had lost a lot of weight by this time. We cared for the shell. There was no person there. We just cared for the body.

Dot: On January 3rd, we took him to see the doctor again. He said: "I really think Stephen should come into hospital", and he was admitted that day. From then on he just seemed to go downhill. The drugs seemed to send him round the bend completely.

Harash: Can you describe his eyes, you know, whether he would be looking at something which wasn't there?

Dot: Two or three times, he said he had looked out of the window and seen a fireman. He also said that he had been up all night because he had been looking after a little boy in the other bedroom. It was nonsense. He would link together things that were not normally connected into one coherent thought in his mind. To you and I, it was nonsense.

I said to the doctor: "There is definitely something adrift here. It's not depression."

The psychiatrist said that he was still of the opinion that Stephen was suffering from deep clinical depression, but he did feel there was a possibility, even a 5% chance, that it could be neurological. He at this stage could not co-ordinate to put food into his mouth.

They took an EEG, but they had great difficulty because Steve thought his head was being sliced off by a saw. So the first EEG they did was useless. They then did two and they were both abnormal. They continued with the drugs and it got to the stage where we said: "Hang on, can we have a second opinion? Nothing seems to be happening."

Stephen by this stage was bad. They had found him in a wardrobe. They could not put him in a room with anybody, because he was being really disruptive, he was moving furniture around, tearing his clothes.

Dave: Sometimes, he could not pick up food with the fork. They were starting to feed him. He was losing weight. They were becoming concerned and started giving him supplements. He had been in four weeks. We had a second opinion in early February. The second opinion was to try him on some new tranquillisers.

Harash: Was he in any way shaking, were there jerky movements in his legs and arms?

Dave: Yes, again that knee tremble was there. Some of the doctors saw this when he was in the hospital, but no one said anything.

Dot: I wouldn't have said he had great difficulty in coordinating things. It was more a case of the shaking. They put his food down with his knife and fork. Three days after later, we found out that they had called the doctor out in an emergency because Stephen had been sitting in the wheelchair at lunchtime, and had put his head back and gone purple. They put him in the bed and all his life signs had gone down. They took blood tests and everything was okay. For all intents and purposes it was considered by the doctors an overdose effect.

Dot: By the evening, he was coming round. He was more or less the way he had been and they said there was no need for concern. The next morning, the doctor rang to say he was sending Stephen over to the neurological unit. Very 'sombre' was the word he used. "He just is not as he would expect him to be."

They took him and eventually got him into the ward under the neurologist. He took Steve off all drugs, absolutely everything.

Dave: The neurologist said: "I think Stephen is suffering from a progressive degenerative disease of the brain". This, obviously, was not something we wanted to hear. We had never heard that term before. Depression we could probably cope with. But this, we were so gob-smacked and so taken aback, we went away disbelieving.

Two or three days later, we had a further meeting with the neurologist, and we said: "Right, we now understand what you're saying. We don't like it, but we hear what you're saying. Can we have a second opinion?"

He said that Stephen was showing such unique symptoms that did not fit any models that he himself would welcome a second opinion. Stephen was transferred to a special unit in London on February 24th, and Stephen was subjected to every test possible. They started with a clean sheet, not accepting anything from neurological unit. They looked again at the MRI and CT scans, which are open to interpretation. They did blood tests, they did lumbar puncture, they did sternum puncture, they did EEGs, ECGs, EMGs, skin biopsy and ultimately the brain biopsy. He had holes everywhere. He had an afternoon with the ophthalmic specialist and it emerged that Stephen could not look up. He could look sideways and down, but not up. That was a very, very distressing afternoon for Stephen and he became very agitated and distressed. He was just terrified, which probably did not give a good quality test. I am sure that happened a lot of times. For example, the EEGs had to be done repeatedly to obtain a good one. Any parent would still have thought it was depression because every time the results came back, they said there was nothing. They had done HIV and that was clear. They had been done so many tests.

We asked to see somebody who deals with psychiatry, and we saw a neuro-psychiatrist. At that stage, Stephen would sit with his eyes shut, but you could prize them open. We did not know whether he was asleep or not. When the neuro-psychiatrist saw him, he was just sitting there, she got no response out of him at all. She said she thought it was a degenerative brain disease. What we saw of the depression at the beginning was him not being able to cope with what was happening, he not understanding what was happening. There was depression there, but she thought that it had all gone and he was not frustrated or frightened any more. He was past that stage, and he was just sitting there.

We asked for a meeting with the neurologist who was giving

the second opinion. She was not very keen to have it. Nobody seemed to be very keen to talk to us all along. She said she was convinced it was a degenerative disease, but they could not put a name to it. It was the operation notes we saw when he went to have his brain biopsy. We noticed from the notes they had left at the end of his bed, they had put 'CJD?' on them. I had wondered about that for a while. All these scary things about cows and the staggering I had seen on the TV, and here we have Stephen. Could it be this, we thought? It was in my mind, but they said they did not know what it was. At that time, the brain biopsy results were still allegedly not available but she did say his life expectancy would be in single years. Steve was getting worse, and no one seemed to be able to help him and he was transferred back to the hospital in Bath, near home.

By then, he was hardly walking because he was ataxic. His balance had certainly gone. His strength had gone because he had not eaten very much, he was very very thin and his legs were just like rubber at times. Sometimes you ended up actually dragging him. He had no physiotherapy, and because I was concerned that he was having no physio and was just sitting or lying in bed, we would get him up. We always made him walk to the toilet, push the wheelchair, just try to do a little bit, but he could hardly walk.

After we got him back at home he wasn't capable of doing anything. Dressing himself, feeding himself, he wouldn't go to the loo, unless somebody says every hour and a half take him to the loo, then he doesn't wet himself, otherwise he does. He just does nothing really, and where does a lad like that live? It's taken until this week to find somewhere that we were happy with and we've ended up with Stephen in a nursing home for the elderly, about ten miles from here, takes us fifteen minutes in the car. Seems to have settled in very well. He's the darling of the Home. We going to take you there to meet him.

Harash: In terms of recognising you and memory, what's that like?

I think until recently he's remembered things from October

back. Things from his childhood are good, but he doesn't remember anything from one minute to the next although he has always remembered us. He has always remembered Helen and he has always remembered people up until recently. We've shown him old photographs and he hasn't recognised his cousins and odd things from the past he doesn't remember. He is getting worse, definitely and he is very drowsy and sleepy now. Whether that's a phase or he's just tired, we don't know. I think that just about brings us up to date.

Dave: One of the things that concerned us at various times was whether Steve was having trouble communicating, or whether he was giving a false impression of his abilities. Was he not communicating for a depressive reason, "I don't want to speak to you, so I'm not going to tell you." Silence does not necessarily mean he does not understand, and silence does not necessarily mean he cannot respond. It just means he is not responding.

Dot: He did respond to younger people far more. When his cousin and his friends visited him he was different. He was talking, putting sentences together, eyes open because it is someone different. He was bored with us.

One day, one of the nurses told us that Stephen had fallen out of bed, over the cot side and cut his eye under his eyebrow. When we walked into the ward, one of the nurses said: "We've never had such a brilliant day with Stephen. He's so bright and alert, and 'with it'." We walked in and there was Stephen in the middle of the ward in his wheelchair with his back to us, and as we walked into the ward they turned the chair round and there was Stephen saying: "Hello mum, hello dad, how are you today?" We had not seen him like that in months. We were absolutely flabbergasted. We had conversations, he put sentences together. He actually cried that day. According to the neurologist in London, he was not capable of any emotion. We asked him whether he wanted to go outside or stay inside. "I want to go outside because its cooler and quiet, and we can talk." He had not said a sentence like that in months. We were really overjoyed. It was the hum of the ward. Everybody was talking about the change. We stayed until about 7 o'clock.

They said at the National that Stephen had lost the ability to pick up but when he got back to Bath, there he was doing it.

They just caught him at a bad time really and you know he has picked tiny little sweets up off my hand with his fingers, like that, and that was weeks after they said that he couldn't do it.

We noticed that he was not as bright the following day. He was still a lot brighter but it gradually tailed off. It was a "coincidence", that was the explanation given. All three of us, all the nursing staff, we were just absolutely gob-smacked. It was so marked. It certainly changed Stephen for those few hours.

Harash: When were you told that Steve might be suffering from CJD?

We only found out it was CJD when we got back to Bath. We saw the consultant who asked whether we understood what they had said in London. We said: "Yes," but there had been no mention of CJD. About a week later, the consultant said he had talked to the neurologist in London and he said: "Of course, she did explain to you that it could be CJD", and we said: "Well, no, she didn't." He said "You must have forgotten."

Of course, I would never have forgotten that. It was uppermost in my thoughts. We were told: "We can't prove anything." CJD was just indicated on the report, which we were not meant to see.

Doctors, well they've all kept asking us, "Has Stephen had blood transfusions abroad and that sort of thing". Could we think of anything? They asked us about whether Steve had growth hormone. I asked what what that was. He's about 5 feet 11 in height. He didn't need growth hormone. Now after talking to you, I think we are reasonably satisfied it's CJD. We don't think they've kept regular records in the hospital of how Stephen was changing and I would have thought that they would have kept a detailed record.

Harash: Well, they do have difficulties. The doctors are being told by the Government and their scientists that nothing has changed so far as CJD is concerned, that BSE is a different disease which won't affect humans, but they are beginning to find that view embarrassing.

That's the impression that we've been given all round, that we would rather not know, we wouldn't want to know but we don't know whether it is political pressure and whether people such as the doctors are told not to publicise it. That is the problem. We do not know how many other young people have the disease.

Harash: Now, what I want you to do is this, tell me as far as you can remember, about Stephen and his diet, the kind of food he ate from as long ago as you remember.

He was always a tall lad at school and very thin but he ate a lot. Mostly, from being five years old to leaving school he had school dinners at lunch time and we believe the last few years they weren't very good. I don't think he had very many of the beefburgers and chips type of food at school. He liked cereals on a morning, porridge, toast that sort of thing. When he was going out with the air training corps he would have a cooked breakfast, sausage, bacon, egg, mushrooms - that sort of thing.

At home, we'd probably have fresh food, non convenience food, two or three times a week. Well, the fresh food if you want to call it that, was very often mince. At home Stephen's favourite meal was roast beef and Yorkshire pudding. We had that maybe once a fortnight, usually on a Sunday. On most weekdays, it would be convenience-type food we bought from supermarkets. As he grew older, he would do a cooked breakfast, which would include a couple of sausages. He was not one for visiting McDonald's and having hamburgers. He liked mince and onion pies. Probably, given his choice, he would plump for sausages and would have sausage and chips once a week. These were probably fairly low-cost beef sausages. We did occasionally have roast lamb, maybe once a month. We've never been pork eaters. Once or twice, we went to a farm and bought fresh meat when we first moved here in 1988. You know, the kind of farm which advertises that they will sell you meat for freezers. They kill their own and chop it, then you buy half of whatever it is and then you bag it and put it in the freezer. I did much the same up North before we moved. I had a friend who opened a butcher's shop in Stockton on Tees and just because they were opening new I went there maybe every six months, and bought maybe £1,500 worth of meat and put it in the chest freezer. That was it really.

We don't like fatty meat so, if I bought a joint, it was rump. If I bought meat to casserole, it was braising steak. We didn't like chops because they were fatty. If I buy mince it was always the best lean mince that they have in the supermarkets. I don't think I bought pork sausages from them. Stephen quite liked sausages. Mind you, we had the best fish and chip shop in the area, people drive ten miles to get to it, about a quarter of a mile down the road and we often went there.

In the past, we used to go regularly for two or three weeks every year to my uncle's farm in Kent, from Stephen being born till he was 14. That was a dairy farm but he didn't have a particularly big herd, about fifty head of cattle.

Harash: Did he have BSE cases on his farm? You know most the farms in Kent did have BSE cases?

Not so far as I know. He stopped dairy farming: well, he died about six or eight years ago and he was a dairy farmer, not a beef farmer.

Harash: So he possibly would have cases of BSE.

Dot: My uncle was very much into farming. He would have one of his animals killed by the local butcher, and we would have fresh-food cooking all the time we were there. Every day there would be a hot meat dish, and most of the time it would be beef from the animal which was killed for us from my uncle's farm. He would get sausages made by this butcher in the village who made good sausages and being a typical farmer's wife, it was all fresh food cooking day in and day out.

We've been racking our brains as you can imagine. One thing that I do remember is Stephen, when he was about four, coming in from playing in the hay loft. He had a tee shirt on and he'd got a piece of straw caught in the inside. It had scratched him and we took the straw out. We didn't think anything more about it until about two weeks later when we were back at Stockton and he got what looked like little warts where these scratches had been. We took him up to the doctors who said: 'Oh, it's a virus' and gave us some cream to rub on. Whether or not that in any way contributed to his becoming ill is something we will never know.

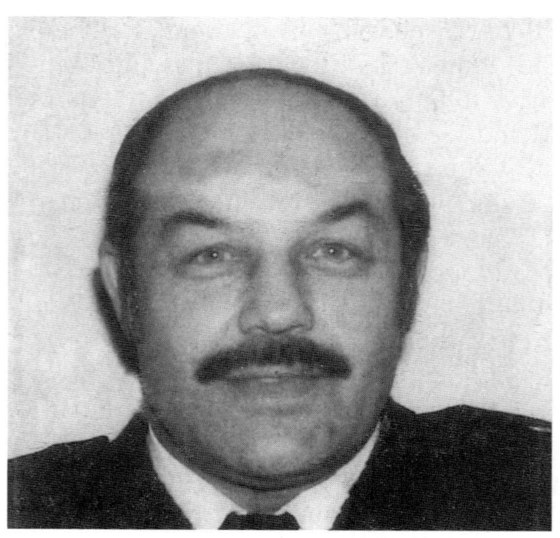

Mike Bowden

Wendy's husband, Mike died at the age of 57 in 1996 after an illness of almost 3 months which began with his complaining of eye trouble and quickly led to his becoming almost blind. This was followed by his having some difficulty and shuffling while walking and developing a tremor in his hands. He was referred by his GP to Hospital where he was found to have a brain tumour but this was discounted as the cause of his illness. Tests continued to be made in the Hospital and, on the 9th of August, Wendy was told that the diagnosis of CJD had been made. Mike left hospital on the 18th August to go home with Wendy. He died on the 24th August, 1996.

In June of 1996, Mike, my husband, was as usual very busy fitting patio doors. It was when he was trying to measure a length of wood for one of the doors, that he complained he couldn't read the measurements. That was the first sign I noticed of anything being amiss. Over the next few days he complained a number of times about his eyesight. His glasses appeared scratched, so I nagged him to visit the Optician and get them changed. The following Friday, he was driving home from his weekly swim and as he passed a row of parked cars, they all appeared to distort in shape and everything he saw appeared as wavy lines. That was enough to make him go to his optician. After an eye examination she told him he wasn't to drive and was to go straight to his G.P. The nightmare had begun.

I arrived home from work about 10 pm that Friday night, and was met by our very distressed daughter Michele who told me that our GP had warned her that there was a possibility of Mike having a brain tumour. This was Friday the 21st June. The next three weeks involved several visits to different hospitals for tests and a brain scan. Nothing showed. By the 12th July, I started leaving meals and sandwiches ready for Mike to eat while we were at work, because if we didn't, he wouldn't eat. He spent most of the day sleeping. Anyone who knows Mike, would know straight away that that was not him at all. There was almost nothing he couldn't turn his hand to.

Mike was now virtually blind. We were told there was very little wrong with his eyesight and it was probably migraine. I even began to believe his eyes weren't as bad as he was making out. This made him very cross and frustrated with me. On the 29th July, I took Mike back to the doctor and pleaded with her to do something and our doctor arranged for him to be seen the next day at Atkinson Morleys Hospital in Wimbledon. They admitted him. After having a MRI, I was almost relieved when a tumour was found at the base of his brain.

The doctor was sure it was a benign growth and in no way life-threatening. Then, finally, they said: "That tumour was a red herring. It couldn't account for the symptoms that Mike was suffering". Dr. Johnson would not perform a biopsy on the tumour because it could be dangerous carrying a risk perhaps of a brain haemorrhage, paralysis or even death. Mike was to remember those words. A barrage of tests were carried out over the next few days: Angiograms, Lumbar Punctures, EEGs. The consultant came to see us and seemed quite excited. He explained that Mike's problem was constant Epileptic fits. He told me that they were going to inject a drug and they were very hopeful that this would give immediate benefits and he would be able to see. He would be cured. I was ecstatic. We went to a special room where Mike was fitted to the EEG machine and the drug was injected into his arm. They gave him more and more.

It was wonderful, the doctor held up two fingers and Mike could see two fingers. More tests were done at the side of his eyes but these he couldn't see. They put him on Epileptic drugs anyway. I had noticed, a few days earlier, when taking Mike for a walk that he was shuffling and I made him walk properly. I now remember he had at the same time a tremor in his hands. On the 6th of August, two of Mike's daughters came down from Scotland. I was supposed to see the Consultant the next day and I waited till the evening but he didn't come.

The 8th of August was a lovely day. Linda, Eileen and Michele took their dad out in the wheelchair and, for a time, he could see everything, even down to the colour of a small leaf on the pavement. He laughed and joked and was in very good spirits. On the 9th of August, the two girls had to return to Scotland. I had another appointment to see the doctor at 2.0 pm.

We arrived at the hospital about 11 am and, when we got to the ward, I could see Mike being walked up and down the ward surrounded by several doctors. He was crying. I moved forward to go to him, but Mike's Consultant held up his hand, telling us to wait. We were in the corridor outside the ward when the doctor came out to us. Linda asked him what was wrong with her dad. He told us Mike had CJD. Both the girls collapsed. The doctor told us that Mike only had months to live. It was awful. We were surrounded by people, there were patients and nurses just a few feet away. We were finally taken to a private room on our own until the girls recovered.

I saw the consultant later and he told us they wanted to do a brain biopsy on Mike. I finally agreed when I was led to believe it was important. The doctors agreed not to tell Mike that this was what they were going to do. As far as he was concerned, it would just be another test and I took him home for the rest of that day. He was so pleased to be home and our four German Shepherd dogs were over the moon to see him.

Mike was able to get around with help and he even managed the stairs that first night. On the Saturday, ever so many people came to see him and I needed to be alone with him to talk. By the Saturday evening, however, he was bad as ever. He was unable to walk even the short distance to the toilet. We slept downstairs that night. It was the Sunday morning when I finally had the chance and the time to talk to him. I told him everything, except for the fact he had CJD. I had to tell him that the disease he had was incurable.

I never ever, want to go through something like that again. A couple of hours later, the hospital phoned asking me to take Mike back. Keith, a very good friend of Mike, offered to take him back in his taxi. That made it easier because he could travel in his wheelchair. We arrived back at the hospital and after settling him in, I told Mike that I would be back in the morning.

Just after 8.0 pm that night the hospital phoned to say Mike was in a very distressed state and would 1 go back. Luckily, another good friend had gone to visit and he had stayed with him until I arrived. Some stupid doctor had told Mike that he was having a brain biopsy in the morning, even though I had given strict instructions that he wasn't to be told. It took a long time to relieve the torture that my husband was going through. I promised him faithfully that I would not now allow them to do the biopsy. He didn't want me to go, because he thought they would come and get him after I had left. When Mike fell asleep, I finally went home. I made sure I was back at 6.30 am.

The anaesthetist came, but I sent him away. The doctor came, and I told him I wasn't allowing the biopsy. When I asked what the chances were that Michael had CJD, I was told that it was more than a 95% chance. To this day, I do not understand why they wanted to perform that biopsy when they knew that, in any event, they could not help or treat him.

I decided to have Mike home. I had been told that he only had a few months to live, and all the family wanted him home. The Social Worker from the hospital was very good. Everything was arranged. The hospital-bed Mike would need, the wheelchair, the ramps and all the rest were provided. On the 18th August Mike came home. He could not see, he could not walk, he could not stand but his sense of humour remained.

On Wednesday, the 21st of August, Michael was admitted into the Phyllis Tuckwell Hospice in Farnham. We have nothing but praise for this wonderful place. Michael died three days later on the 24th August 1996.

My family and I suffered continuous anguish throughout the whole of Mike's illness which has left a scar we will never lose. We hate to think anyone else should have to endure what we experienced.

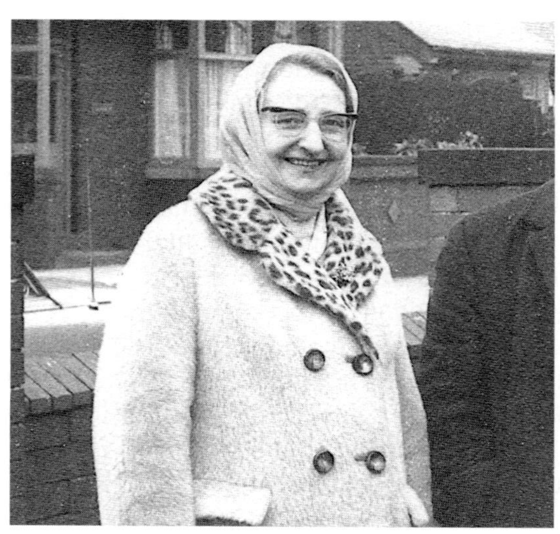

Ivy Tattersley

After an illness of some four months from the symptoms first appearing, Ivy died in 1992 at the age of 72. Starting at Christmas, her family noticed that her memory was failing and she was frequently lapsing into short periods of sleep. A few weeks later, she developed a tremor in her hands and was seen by her GP. He took the view that she was suffering from Alzheimer's. Only her sister-in law's insistence led to Ivy being seen by a neurosurgeon who recognised that she was seriously ill and admitted her to hospital. His first suspicion was that she had a brain tumour but later revised his opinion and told her family that she CJD. Six weeks later, she died.

She was a gents hairdresser. She was always healthy strong woman, a very strong woman. I used to envy her because, when we went out and took some bread with us to feed the ducks, she could bend down to feed them and I couldn't. She was full of energy and go, right up to her starting to be ill. She didn't get married until she was about forty five.

I didn't notice anything the matter with Ivy until about Christmas time. She worked for us on a market stall. She could add things up straight away, she had always been very quick but she started getting unsure about costs and prices and adding up. My daughter in law noticed that and said: "I see Ivy's beginning to slow down. She was always so sharp at adding up."

Coming nearer to the Christmas time, she was just feeling not too good and I suggested that she should have a holiday. I suggested that she went to stay with her brother at Derby and felt that that might do her a bit good. She didn't want to go there any more, she said. I also noticed that, to begin with, she would come to me every night and sit beside me but then just dose off. We'd be watching the TV and I kept nudging her and saying: "Ivy, you're missing the TV." She'd start laughing at me and a few minutes later she'd be back to sleep again. There was something not right. I asked her to go to the doctors. She went to the doctors and he just said that it was, "Oh Lord, it's something to do with her heart again." He gave her some tablets, but they didn't do any good. I said: "It's nothing to do with your heart, Ivy", and told her, "If you wouldn't mind, I will go with you to the doctors. Tell him I'll pay for you to see a specialist, if he'll give you a letter." He would not give her a letter.

She only lived six weeks after him telling us what was wrong with her. She just deteriorated so rapid. She died on the 16th April, so she'd not been getting forgetful for long but I do remember one thing that happened, probably twelve months or so before all her trouble began. Its only a silly little thing, but I have thought about it many a time since. We were having a tea party in the church hall and Ivy was selling some raffle tickets and Father Mace wanted to say grace. She would insist on going on selling these raffle tickets and Father Mace kept trying to tell her to come and sit down. It seemed she didn't grasp what was going on. At the time, I thought it was just a bit of stupidness.

So, I went to the doctors with her and he was furious. He slung his stethoscope across the room onto a bed and he raged at me. He said: "You think I wear this for a necklace? Who's the Doctor here?" I said: "No, I don't think it's an ornament. You're the Doctor, doctor. I am just very worried about my sister- in-law. She is not well. Her speech keeps going slurred."

He said: "She's not had a stroke". I said: "I never thought for one minute that she has had a stroke, but I'm worried about her." He said: "She's senile." She had Alzheimer's disease. I just don't know, because she had started all of a sudden to be feeling poorly. Oh, he was treating her for angina, and I was sure it was not angina. That doctor, I don't think he was even interested. When he mention her being senile, I said: "Never in this wide world doctor. She worked for us on a busy market, adding up, taking money, giving change right up to Christmas and this is only the first week in February.

No, she's not senile. Could I have a letter for her to see a specialist?" He said: "No." Anyway, that was on a Thursday. The following Monday I was so worried about her that I rang a friend of mine and I said to her, "Jean, do you know of a brain surgeon." She said: "Yes, I know one in Sheffield". She told me the number and I rang this brain surgeon up and asked for an appointment. They said: "Yes, but I would have to have a letter from her doctor." So, I sent her husband and Pauline, my daughter, back to the doctor's, but he wouldn't give them a letter. They had it out with him and he told them to come back the next day and they finally did get a letter, but it wasn't what I'd asked for. I went with her to see this neurosurgeon, when we got an appointment. It was at four o'clock, Saturday afternoon. By then, her hand was going funny and shaking. That had started before the specialist saw her. Her hand was trembling and I had got her a ball to squeeze and I kept telling her to squeeze it and I kept rubbing her arm. I think people thought that I was getting a bit overprotective towards her.

Well, we all noticed it. I'll give you one example. Just before she went into hospital I remember she was downstairs and she wanted to go to the toilet upstairs. Her brother was over at the time. He said to me "You ought to see her up those stairs." I had to laugh because, although it was a steep staircase, she just ran up that staircase like that, no hesitation whatsoever. She just flew up that staircase and that was just before she went into hospital. Before she went into hospital she was in bed at home for about a week. I used to go in each morning to see to her and, mentally, she was deteriorating every day. It was her mental deteriorating that was the fastest. Definitely. She was perfectly normal otherwise, just as she'd always been, and that's what made me think she'd got a brain tumour. It is difficult to explain, but, if you spoke to her, she wasn't with you. I think the first thing I noticed was that she was looking at me and it frightened me to death when she did that.

I told the doctor what I'd noticed. I said: "Her speech is going slurred, sometimes she is looking at me and I don't think she sees me. I just have a funny feeling about her. I think she looks sometimes as if her mind's blank." Her husband were annoyed and swore at me for saying these things. Doctor told him to shut up and let me tell him. He examined her and then he told us afterwards that she was seriously ill and that he was admitting her immediately into the Alanchurch Hospital. There, a nurse pulled the curtain round and I heard my sister-in- law say to the nurse, "I'm dying nurse, I'm dying." That upset me terrible. I said to the doctor, "What do you think is wrong with Ivy." He said: "Well I don't really know, but we've got to find out. She could have had a stroke, but I don't think so." I asked him, "What else could she have." He said: "Well, she could have a brain tumour." I said: "Well, that is what I've been worried about, that she's got a brain tumour, that's what I'm frightened of." The following Sunday the doctor wanted to see us. He'd found out what was wrong. She had deteriorated rapidly.

I think there was two different doctors and they were giving her tablets and things, you know, but nothing was doing her any good. I got in touch with my own daughter, and asked her to come down and take Aunt Ivy and me for a run out. I says: "Lets see if we can get these drugs blown out of her body, because they're not doing her a bit of good. I would like her to get a bit of fresh air and see if it bucks her up a bit." We took her out and I can remember her sitting at the table, just eating while her eyes were just vacant. Even though her husband said I was crackers. Nobody would believe me when I said that about Ivy, "She's looking at us but she's not looking at me. Somehow, she's looking at me but she's not seeing it's me." When I went with her to the doctors, he wouldn't have it at all. I never ever went back to that doctors, and I've always regretted not going back and telling him what I thought about him. What annoyed me was the fact that when I told him her speech was slurred, he should have done something about it, and I do think it was his job to try to find out what was wrong with her.

Well, she started having terrible shakes in her hands and legs in the hospital and she had been in with these other patients but then they put her into a room of her own and barrier nursed her.

I'll never forget, because when I went, I heard this terrible noise and, oh, it frightened me to death. She was just shaking all over, shaking dreadful. I tried to hold her legs to rub but she'd lost her feelings. By that time, she didn't know anything.

Suddenly, one day, the doctor said that she had Jacobs Creutzfeldt Syndrome, but we'd never ever heard of that, neither had anybody else. Nobody knew what to make of it. They were all making fun of mad cow disease, you know. We didn't know anything about it. One day, two or three years later, my son brought me the Yorkshire Post and there on the front page there was a piece, about so big, in the middle of the front page. I think I still have it because I cut it out. It said something about children in America having been given growth hormone and it said that they'd stopped that treatment because some of the children had developed CJD. Ivy was ill only from Christmas to the middle of April.

I can tell you this for certain - and I know when it happened, because my granddaughter got married at the beginning of January — she told another daughter in law of mine, she said: "Brenda, I'm dying." She didn't tell me, I know, because she knew I'd be upset and worried. Yes, that was in the January. She said: "Brenda, I'm dying." She did not know why she was dying, there appeared to be so little wrong with her, and none of us would have thought that she was dying. It was just like these periods you have when you're off colour but you pull yourself round. It was just like that at first.

From February, I had to help her to dress. She just went rapidly downhill. I'll tell you one incident with her in the hospital. There were four beds in an open ward. She wanted to go to the toilet and she had gone to the toilet. I had wanted to go in with her but the nurse said: "No, she'd go herself." Anyway, they couldn't get her out and they tried and she spread herself with the wall and they could not get her out of that toilet. Well, I knew Ivy and I understood her. I kept saying to them "Excuse me, could I help." They told me I was interfering and to get out of the way. In the end they fetched a door joiner to take the door jamb out, but they still couldn't get her out. I begged them, "Please let me go and talk to her." In the end they just said: "Oh, go and see what you can do." I went in and the only thing she wanted to do was to wash her hands before she came out of the toilet and they weren't letting her do it. She washed her hands and she folded the towel up so carefully, smoothly and carefully, and hung it on the towel rail and just walked out.

Harash: Could she count at this stage?

I don't think she could have counted. She could not feed herself. I went every day and used to feed her. I think she'd had the best appetite in the hospital at first and then I noticed it gradually getting less and less until she wasn't eating at all. I said to a young nurse, "If I was you, I wouldn't bother to bring the meals into her because she's not eating them and its a shame to waste good food. She's not touching it at all." She says "Oh, I'll make her have it." She put these things round her but she still could not make her take a spoonful. So, after that they did it with a tube. For the last three weeks, I would say she was in a coma. I didn't stay with her as long as I had done once she started going into the coma because I couldn't. It was too distressing to be there, just to see her lying there. The only time that her husband showed any interest in her was when she was in the coma and we knew she was going to die.

I'd noticed there was some water on the floor and I asked the nurse if Ivy had done that and she said: "Yes". I said she's losing control of her bladder. I remember my son going to see her. The last time I ever heard her say anything was when she put her arms around him and said: "Hard." They call him Howard: she couldn't say Howard, but I could tell what it was she had said. So, she could recognise people. That was until she went into a coma. She knew when we'd gone, for all she was losing her speech and I'll tell you something else, I knew, right from the start, she couldn't have read anything about her kind of illness.

She did have false teeth, but not mouth ulcers or anything like that. I can remember her getting badly scratched. She was an animal lover, a very big animal lover. Well, I can always remember. She always used to sit with her legs parted and I could see all all these scratches down her legs. One day, I just said to her for a bit of fun like, "What's Joe been doing to you Ivy. I can see all your legs scratched Ivy. What's gone wrong." She said that her black cat - and it was devil - it wasn't a cat that you could stroke, had jumped on her while she was dressing her other cat on her knee and scrawled all down her legs.

She used to buy ox liver and things like that for her cats. She'd often buy a pound of what they called offal, though I don't really know what was in it, and cook it for them. She'd stir it up with gravy and biscuits. The cats, she used to buy ox liver for them and cook it or get them chicken or mince, served up with gravy and biscuits. It was usually things like liver, offal, she used to buy for them.

Harash: You said that she used to make broth with sheep's head. Did she ever use cows brains?

I think it would be just sheep. I will tell you something about that. My husband was a beef and pork butcher by trade.

Harash: Oh, you didn't tell me that, its very important.

He was a beef and pork butcher from leaving school and he learned the trade but we had the market stall. We had a snack bar, and we used to sell pies and peas. We used to make our own pies. Now, through the war, meat was rationed but we could get cows heads, you know, ox heads, they were free from ration. We got those. You could cut the beast's cheek off it and it was nice meat that. Occasionally, I have known him chop them in two and get the brains out.

Harash: What would he use the brains for?

It used to be considered a luxury at one time, didn't it. I never ate any. My mother would have had some and my husband would certainly have had some. Yes, Ivy would have had some.

Harash: Would you know how they cooked them?

They could fry or toast them, or have them with gravy or something like that. We just cooked it, we boiled the meat, minced it and mixed it with biscuit, seasoned it and put it into the pies. Now, in Scotland, they used the brains as well in these meat pies. My husband did not always get the brains out because he had to chop the head in two to do it, and that was a bit laborious. That was the only reason we didn't do it.

Harash: You told me that Ivy, had had dogs and cats. If she was eating brains, would she feed the dogs with it?

Well that I don't know, but she'd definitely give the dogs anything that was left over, possibly raw, before she cooked it.

Harash: You said she didn't marry until she was forty five. So, if she was making broth with sheeps heads, who would split the heads for her?

She would get the butcher to do it. She wouldn't do it herself. It was a family butchers, they knew one another. You see, butchers have what they call cleavers. They just give one sharp tap with one when they know the job, just one tap and the head just splits. I'll tell you something else. Funnily enough, her mother's sister who lives at Dewsbury, they were always having sheep's head broth because Aunt Elsie, when she used to come, she'd always be talking about having had sheep's head broth. She used to love it. Now, Pauline, my stepdaughter, tells me that, when she was brought up with them, they had sheep's head broth every week. Well, it was easy and cheap to make. They'd just wash the head and it would be chopped, you know, cut through the middle. Then they'd cook it with vegetables, things like that. Pauline said they'd have it about once a week because they loved it.

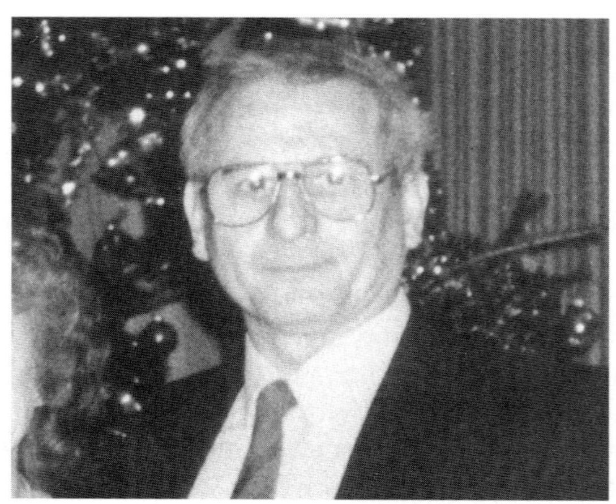

Len Franklin

Len Franklin of York, a driver, who had also worked in an abattoir for a number of years, died from CJD at the age of 53 in 1996. As a hobby, he often brought home beasts' heads, removed the horns and then carved them. The first sign of trouble was when, while driving on familiar roads, he became confused and was unable to appreciate where he was. During the following 9 months of his illness, he aged rapidly. His partner of six years, Pat Broadhead, nursed him almost continuously at home throughout his illness.

It was she who contacted the author, Harash Narang, and invited him to test Len by his live urine test for CJD. That urine test was performed a month before Len's death and was found to be positive for CJD.

Shortly before his death, Pat told Harash the history of Len's illness and how it had affected their two lives and how she was alerted to the possibility that Len's illness was akin to that of the cows with BSE she saw on her TV. The symptoms which Pat described are typical of Narang Disease. A month later, Len died. Following his death, a post-mortem was done which, at Pat's request, Harash attended. The result of this Post-mortem was to confirm that Len had died from CJD. Further examination of his brain led Harash to confirm Len had died from Narang Disease (new variant).

When I met Len six years ago he worked for Polar. He valeted cars and had to deliver and collect them. The first inclination of anything being amiss was at the end of August, 1995 at the end of my holiday - Len couldn't go because he was working - when he was to travel to Basingstoke to pick me up. At 9 o'clock in the evening he rang to say: "Hello darling I'll be with you in about half an hour, I'm only a few miles away". At one o'clock in the morning, he still hadn't arrived. We got another telephone call from him but that didn't make sense at all and my son-in-law went out to search for him. He found him not very far from the house, walking in the opposite direction, utterly confused. At that time we joked with him and made fun saying: "It's only you that could get lost". He was very tired but we put that down to his having been driving all day. He did complain of a headache and that was unlike him. In all the five years we'd been together he'd never complained of anything at all.

The next day he seemed OK, at least until we were travelling back to York, when he got utterly confused again. I wasn't really concerned, really didn't think anything about it - mind you, we finished up going through the middle of London. I was reading the map. If I said turn right, he turned left and if said turn left, he turned right. It still didn't strike home to me that anything was seriously amiss.

We finally arrived home that night having taken about four hours longer than we should have. Len was extremely tired, but that was all. He didn't say that there was anything wrong with him. On another occasion, either shortly before or after that, he had been working - again driving - and he came on to me and said: "Something very strange happened to me today. I was driving the vehicle" - and I think he was going to London again - "and my mind suddenly left me and I didn't know where I was going, I didn't know why I was going and even whose vehicle it was. I had to pull up at the side of the road and it took me about half an hour to get my head together."

Luckily, he had had all his papers on the dashboard anyway and when he got his head together, he was able to carry on his journey. He had been utterly confused and lost. From then on, it seemed to be a steady decline. He complained of being tired all the time and aching in his back. He did suffer from a frozen shoulder at times, so that didn't surprise me. One morning he got up and said he felt very funny as though his head didn't belong to him. He went on like that for a few days but he was still working. At the same time he started with a funny little dry cough. He was a smoker, so again we didn't worry unduly about that. He was coughing up mucous and I told him he really should see the doctor. He said: "It's because of my ciggies".

That took us into September 1995 when he started having slight memory losses. For five years I've had the same day off work each week and he couldn't hack it. He kept asking: "Are you working today?" I said: "No, it's my day off". "Oh, I forgot". Little things like that.

His co-ordination started going - thinking back, I feel dreadful about it now. He used to sit in the chair and flick his ash. Instead of putting it in the ashtray, he'd just flick it anywhere, or he'd throw things into the waste bin and they'd finish up at the other side of the room. I thought he was just being silly so I told him off- I said to him: "It's like living in a bar room."

His memory losses and confusion increased- they seemed to come and go - and then he started weaving about. It was very slight at first. He started veering off slightly. This became more and more noticeable and he would say: "I don't know what's wrong with me." His hands started shaking but only very slightly. He lost interest in a lot of things and seemed depressed. He would sit there gazing into space. I used to say: "What's the matter love?" He'd say "I don't know, maybe it's the weather." It was not like him - he was always whistling or singing. His lack of co-ordination got worse and worse and more and more noticeable. It was as though he'd had one drink too many. At this stage, I insisted he went to the doctor's. He went and the doctor told him he'd got a virus - there was a virus going round - and that it would take about six weeks to clear up. He was given some tablets to take. He took them for about three weeks but his co-ordination got worse and worse. His speech started to slur as though he was drunk. Not all the time - it was spasmodic.

I insisted he go back to the doctor's because his tablets weren't doing him any good. It was a locum, and she told him to continue with the tablets and to come back when his own doctor was there. I was very annoyed about this. I said to the doctor: "There is something seriously wrong with him and he wants sorting and I want him in hospital for observation." So they did take him in for a 24 hour observation in the City Hospital in the Neurology ward. But that wasn't until Oct 25th and, all the time, he was having all these problems. I couldn't' believe they were only going to have him in for such a short time - I couldn't see what they could observe in 24 hours.

I visited him in the morning of 26th. They had told him they were releasing him in the afternoon. I said: "Will you please ring me and let me know and I'll get a car organised to pick him up." I waited in till about 2 pm and I rang the hospital. They said: "He's gone". They'd released him and I couldn't believe it. So I said: "I asked you to ring me" and they said: "He said he was all right, he would manage on his own."

I was told by the head nurse that, if I went to the District Hospital, we'd find him there because they'd sent him there for an X-ray and some blood tests. We went there but couldn't find him. He eventually got home about 5.30 in the evening, absolutely shattered, worn out. He was struggling to walk. It was as though he was drunk, really drunk and he'd lost his direction again. He came in, sat on the settee and he looked really awful. He had walked all the way home and that's quite a distance. It takes me half an hour walking briskly. He'd been to the hospital as well, but I didn't find out until later that he'd forgotten to have one of the tests done. I just couldn't believe that they let him out like that. He came home on 26th October and from then on he became steadily worse.

On the 31st October he saw the doctor again because his co-ordination was getting worse and his hands were shaking more noticeably by then and, on November 8th, he went in for an EEG. On 13th Nov he had a head scan and, in my ignorance, I thought it was going to be a deep head scan and would show up whatever was the trouble but it showed up nothing.

His walking got worse. He'd get up from the settee and get his legs going, but only with difficulty. I remember one day he started running, and he ran across the room really fast and he couldn't stop and, if I hadn't been in his way with my son, he'd have gone through the window. He knocked us over, he was going so fast. On 20 November he went back to hospital again. I'd taken him down for the results of his scan and he wanted to walk and it was a long way. It took us ages. When he was walking, he said he wanted to walk on the road because he thought the buildings were going to fall in on him. He was lifting his feet up as though walking up steps when he was only on the pavement. I took him in to see the Neurologist for the results of the test. He said the head scan showed clear. I said: "Well, I don't understand that because there is something obviously wrong with the part of the brain which gives him co-ordination."

The neurologist gave him tests - touch his nose and things like that and he was well off target. He went round the back of his head somewhere and the neurologist said: "Well, there's obviously something very wrong with the cerebellum. That's the part of the brain that gives him his co-ordination". He told me to take Len home and that he would get him back into hospital again. His walking was so erratic and so dreadful that the nurse said: "There's no way can this man walk out of here." She rang up and said it was an emergency and she wanted a bed straight away for him. He was to be admitted into City Hospital, into the neurology department.

I brought him home in a taxi, got him ready and took him to the City Hospital. He walked into the hospital and, during the first few days, he went through various tests including blood tests but they all showed up negative. I had had to get for them a list of chemicals which he used at work to clean cars.

His walking got worse. On November 27 he went for an ultrasound on his tummy and the only thing they found was that he had a couple of gallstones in his gall bladder. On 30 November, he had a broncholopscopy. I was told the tests were clear apart from the gallstones. He was still moving around for himself, although with great difficulty and his co-ordination was quickly getting worse and worse. He fell three times while he was in hospital and injured his ankle - once going over the edge of a carpet and once out of his wheelchair and the other time he'd gone over the side of his bed.

I remember reading the daily notes at the bottom of his bed on one occasion and there were strict instructions in them that he was to be watched at all times. I couldn't understand how they could be letting him fall out of a wheelchair. He was shaking at that time, his movements were jerky ... like automated. He was still saying: "I wish they'd hurry up and find out what is wrong with me and then I can go home and get back to work." He was still, at times, completely clear in his thoughts and knew what he wanted. His memory loss was intermittent. He would have good days and bad days. He just wanted to come home and he kept packing his bags - he packed them about four times a day.

By December, he was put into a wheelchair and getting more confused. There were remissions between the periods of confusion but each time the waves were getting shorter. My son had been talking to a psychiatrist friend who advised him to prepare me for the worst as he thought it could be CJD. We had read about cases of that disease in the papers and knew what it might mean. On December 11th we saw the doctor who told us that nothing had shown up on the tests. We then asked him whether it could in fact be CJD. He said: "Yes, that's at the top of our list". That was just the duty doctor on the ward. He did say there was a possibility it was a cancer which hadn't shown up but whatever it was, Len was a very seriously ill man and he hadn't got long to live. I knew the disease but I didn't realise the short time - they thought he only had months - and not very many at that. They had ruled every other illness out. They had given him every possible test. They had sent him to Hull for another MRI scan - I can't remember the day that was. There's a few days missing out of my diary because I was so distraught.

Harash: Did you mention his having worked at the abattoir?

Yes. On 22nd December, Dr Will from the CJD Surveillance Unit in Edinburgh came to see us and asked us all about Len's lifestyle - what type of work Len had been involved with, what kinds of food did he eat, how much did he drink and how much did he smoke. He didn't ask any leading questions. He would know Len worked in an abattoir because I put that down on a list for the hospital. He said that the usual span from the onset to finish was six months. That we already expected from what Simon's psychiatrist friends had told us. Dr Will kept saying he wasn't a medical man, he was a neurologist.

Harash: What did he mean by that?

Pat: I don't really know. I did ask Dr. Will: "Will Len go deaf and blind and find it difficult to swallow?". He said: "Yes".

Harash: Did you ask him, how Len had got CJD from?

Pat: He did tell us that there was a theory that it was hereditary and asked whether any other relatives of Len's had died and what they had died from. My only concern at that time was Len, I didn't care about anybody else.

Len at this stage still wanted to come home. He wasn't talking properly; his sentences were short and he spoke haltingly. He couldn't remember the names; he forgot my name. Oh yes, he always used to say: "Hello love I'm glad you're here." He laughed when he couldn't remember my name. He said: "Aren't I stupid. I can't even remember my wife's name?"

I asked you (Harash) to do a urine test for CJD and you told me it was positive when we met in London on April 16th, 1996.

Harash: Let me go over two or three things. When did you first observe he was shaking?

Pat: The back end of August, 1995 but it was only very slight at first, just like a tremble. As his co-ordination got worse, he found it increasingly difficult to walk in a straight line. When he could walk, there was something wrong with him because he'd veer slightly to the right or to the left. He'd be going through a door and maybe just bump himself. When he was driving he was weaving about and going to the centre of the road. That was pretty frightening, but he didn't know he was doing it. I'd say pull over and he'd say: "I'm all right".

He was feeding the dogs one night and he was spilling their food all over the floor and not managing to put it in their dishes. He was still managing to feed himself all right. He wasn't dribbling his food because he kept his mouth close to the plate. He was always a fast eater. Len was forgetting names. He still had a sense of humour. I went out and bought a badge with my name on and I went back to the hospital and I said: "I've got something funny here, Len" He said: "What?" I said: "I've got a badge with my name." He said "I know your name - it's Pat."

He came out of hospital on Dec 23rd. He was still managing to get to the toilet. He would go in his wheelchair or if someone walked him. He was still managing to clean his teeth and wash his face, but that quickly got beyond him. He couldn't shave anymore because he kept cutting himself. I used to do it for him. When he got home, he said to me he wasn't going to go back into hospital and I was to ring the nurse and tell her.

He did not know what was wrong with him. All this time, he just kept saying he wanted to get better and get back to work and get the house done up. He wanted to go straight to the pub for a pint, so Simon took him. He recognised his sister and called her by her name. He was extremely happy to be home and slept until 6 o'clock that night after his drinkiepoos. He sat and watched TV and nattered to everybody as best he could.

He started making very weird noises which terrified me in the night. He wasn't calling names and shouting. He was just making the most horrible weird noises and - I never told this to anyone else - but while I was lying there listening to him .. it just sounded like cattle. Like the bellowing of a cow. I wrote it in my diary and it would go on and on until he fell asleep.

He was still very loving at that time. He wanted his cuddles. He said that when he came home he didn't want to sleep in a bed on his own. He wanted to come back into the big bed and be with me. He couldn't wash himself or do anything for himself at that time. I had to wash him and do everything for him. He laughed a lot at the things he saw. He did start hallucinating. He was always doing things with his hands. He started pulling at his clothes, grasping at his clothes all the time and reaching out with his hands all the time. I said: "What are you doing Len?"

He said: "I'm making guns, I'm making guns." He started moving his hands about and I said: "What are you doing now, sweetheart?" He said: "I'm firing guns, I'm firing guns."

Another time he was looking up and he was moving about with his arms out and making funny noises and I asked him what he was doing... It was all very distressing because at times I didn't know what to do for the best, but I thought the best thing to do was humour him and join him in whatever he was doing. He said I'm riding this spaceship - Starship Enterprise - and he was going round. He said: "I'm going to land it up there" and it was the top of the curtain rail he pointed to. He did all the actions and he landed this spaceship safely. I said: "Well next time you go off, can I go with you?" He asked me where I would like to go and so I said: "Well, you know, Cyprus. Well, I've never been to Cyprus. Take me there and tell me all about it." So he told me: "Get in and fasten your belt." He took me round Cyprus and showed me the sights. Before he became ill, if he had any problems he would never talk about them. He'd keep them to himself and maybe go off in a huff and then come back later. Simon was trying to get to know how he felt about things. His feelings and his fears. He told him he wanted to go back and live in Cyprus - he had always loved it there.

He did make one strange comment on December 24th, Christmas Eve. I told him my sister had rung and he said: "Have you told her that I've got one foot in the grave?" That's the only inclination he gave of knowing how ill he was. He was just home for a few days when I realised he had a thrombosis in his leg. I had to fight - and let him enjoy his Christmas at home. He had a good meal and everything and then he went back into hospital for his thrombosis and he was in there a week and he deteriorated very badly that week. He could still move around in his bed - he had cot sides on. How he got to the bottom of the cot we don't know, but we often used to find him with his legs hanging out. He just wanted to get out of "the cage" as he called it. At that time I could manage to turn him around. He would still speak to people on the ward, and he did as best he could. He would ask for fish and chips. He could still make decisions for himself. It was getting through to us how ill he was because we could see how badly his speech was affected.

On January 5th, the neurologist asked our permission to record a video of him doing a test and I agreed. Len went through the tests with flying colours. He remembered all the days of the week, months of the year and a couple of other simple little questions they asked him. His only problem was co-ordination - touching his nose or touching the doctor's hands. He'd taken his glasses off. He said he didn't need them anymore. He took his watch off - he said he didn't need that anymore. He could still tell the time. I used to hold fingers up and he would count them. After a week, he came home and after his first day at home he'd lost movement in his legs altogether. He couldn't hold his body weight on them. I had great difficulty in the first couple of days getting him to the toilet or to his commode. He was having a struggle to use his bowels. He thinks he wants to go but his brain's not telling him when and where. He needed a convene fitted because he didn't have control over his urine.

It was all very distressing because in the end it all came down to money. When they'd given him 48 hours to live, I asked for two sleepovers from the Goldsborough people and the next day the social services woman came in. She never even looked at him - she said: "Oh, I've had the report. Len's a bit better today, you don't need anybody to sleep over tonight. I've got to go and try to find the money for the last two nights you've had".

Len was still making comments - things like, "that tea smelt good". He still had sexual inclinations in January which I found very surprising. He said he wanted to love me and things like that - he was still able to get aroused. He understood a joke. He always did have a sense of humour, right up to a week before he died.

Harash: Had Len ever been a blood donor?

"I very much doubt it. He was frightened of needles. His teeth were bad. He had fillings broken and worn down and he still wouldn't go to the dentist. He did start having a skin complaint at the back of his legs - they went all red and itchy. He used to be scratch, scratching them - that would be about August 1994.

Harash: How long did he work in abattoir?

He worked there for about 18 months, as far as I know. He looked after the animals.

Harash: Did you know about his bringing heads home and about him taking out the horns and carving them? Did he work at the abattoir before he met you?

Pat: Yes: about two years before.

Harash: Would he bring meat from the abattoir.

Pat: He would eat a lot of convenience food, pies and things, probably buy a steak pie. He used to love beef and they used to get a lot of beef from the abattoir. He once got some here. He went playing pool one night and he came back with a big carrier full of beef joints that he bought from a friend who worked at the abattoir. He had bumped into him in the pub and he got this beef. It was one huge piece and Len cut it up into about 8 joints - that would be about 2 years ago.

Harash: When he became ill, did you see him age very quickly in terms of appearance?

Pat: Yes, as he got further into the illness, he did seem to age very quickly. His face looked drawn. His eyes seemed to sink in. He was about 13 stone with a lovely physique. He was a manual worker and he was really strong. But in the end I could lift him, and turn him over physically on my own. I think he only weighed about 7st. His throat had been closing up gradually throughout January and into February and he was down to just two or three spoonfuls of Weetabix. Fluids he could manage, but not solid food. I could just get things like rice pudding down him but even then I had to dilute them with milk. I got a blender to blend foods for him, but he couldn't even take that really. So I went onto baby foods. His throat was just full of mucous - he would cough it up, but he couldn't spit it out. His mouth and windpipe was full of it. I had to keep pumping it out every 10 or 15 minutes - day and night - to stop him choking.

He died on 28th Feb, 1996 and, all the time, I had nursed him at home. At least I could give him what he wanted. You, yourself came to see me about a week before his death.

Harash: What was the most difficult thing for you when you were looking after him?

Pat: I think suctioning him out - I'd been given no help - nobody had said we can use this on him or we can use that on him. I'd even gone through the kitchen looking for something. I'd thought about using a tube which I had to suck fat off gravy. Then, I had to call in a nurse one night for his bed sores. Straight away she said: "Haven't you got a suction? I can't believe you haven't got one." I got one the very next day. The nursing sister had been coming in every day - she had never mentioned it.

Harash: Do you think that's the kind of experience anyone should have?

Pat: I think the answer to that is that I loved Len and I knew he didn't want to be in a hospital and if you love somebody you do everything you can to help them. There was no way I could have seen Len be in hospital without the love and care and attention he deserved and that's what he got. I loved him. If I was ill, I wouldn't want somebody to shove me in another place, or another home, away from all my loved ones. All the time he was in hospital, he kept packing his bags four times a day. He wanted to come home. It's so impersonal in hospital. They are very good and they give you all the care they can, but Len would have been lucky if he had got a pat on the head twice a day when they passed him.

Harash: You told me you had difficulty getting morale support. Do you think you, yourself, are now in a good position to give advice and help?

I'm no expert, but I think l am more of an expert than any of the nurses in the hospital. There was nothing they gave Len, nothing they could give him, they didn't give him any medication whatsoever.

Harash: Did you try to prolong his life in any way?

Pat: I shortened his life by not having him intravenously fed. I was given the choice. The doctors all had different opinions. One said if he goes into dehydration, it's very, very distressing and, to lessen that, you should have him put into hospital and fed intravenously. I said: "What for?" Another one was more sympathetic and said he agreed with me entirely. "Do not prolong his life, because he hasn't got a life. He's going to die anyway." He said: "If we take him in for the chest infection, he's going to be hooked up to God knows how many machines. Then, if we get him clear of that, he's only going to die in a couple of weeks with it anyway, because it will start up again."

So I decided that Len had suffered enough and, although it broke my heart, when he was taking less and less fluid, maybe one ounce of fluid a day, I had to sit and watch him die. That was a very difficult thing to do and I think that that's what's mainly distressing me now although, in retrospect, I know it was the best thing for Len. But he wasn't suffering. I think at the end he knew himself how near the end he was, because, when I was trying to get fluids down him, he would turn his face away from me as if to say: "No, darling don't, don't do it anymore." He would close his teeth tight.

Harash: Tell me what sort of morale support do you think was needed and what would you have found helpful?.

Pat: Basically, just someone to talk to. I did ring Sandra Galloway. Somebody gave me her number, and I rang her when Len was first diagnosed. She told me she was sorry to hear about it and would keep in contact with me, but she never did. So, I didn't bother ringing her again. There was nobody. You were the only one who was here within a few hours of a phone call and, since then, you have helped me understand what was happening and supported me all the way. In fact, Frances, Peter Hall's mother, rang me quite a few times here. She told me you asked her to do so. But it's really someone to talk to, even if it's only to swap symptoms or talk about what you were going through. But there's was nobody till I phoned you. One or two of the other girls from your office phoned and gave me a lot of moral support.

Harash: At the end, when he died, what happened then?

Pat: For the last week of his life, he hadn't had any food or drink. He was just lying there. Nobody told me what would happen if he went into a coma. None of the nursing staff that we had been in touch with - nobody explained anything to me. Len weed on me, excreted on me. I actually had his mouth fluids and his mucous on my mouth when I was kissing him one night and he coughed and I had it stuck all over me. I even used the same spoon as him. And yet, the funeral parlour man wouldn't even let me see him. He would be too infectious, he said.

I asked: "Will he go into a coma? Is he in a coma?"

"No, he's just peaceful. We think he was still hearing" they said.

Whether he was seeing, I'm not sure. He used to look at you vacantly, but I like to think he could still see. Although he wasn't taking food, I did still manage to get some medication down him. I said to him: "Open your mouth, Darling." Whether he heard me or couldn't co-ordinate his mouth movements to my request, I don't know. Sometimes, when I was cleaning his mouth out, his jaw would close and he couldn't open it straightaway voluntarily. But I did notice, if I went forward towards him with a spoon, his little mouth would open like a blackbird, so he could see. I'm positive he could, although he'd no co-ordination over his eye movements. For about two days before he died, maybe longer, he could still feel pain. I know that because he had his bowels vacated a couple of times and he whinged and moaned - didn't like it, so I know he felt pain. He went a funny colour and he was cold. His feet were like ice and yet at the same time his body clock had gone all wrong. His head, his cheeks and his face were hot, he was sweating and yet, his little feet were freezing. That was two or three days before he died. He looked just like a skeleton with skin stretched over.

Harash: Tell me, Pat, did anyone tell you that if he did die, there was a number you should phone, someone you could contact for help?

Pat: No. I was just left to my own devices. I was very frightened as well. Nobody told me that the police would come.

Harash: What do you mean that the police would come?

Pat: He died about half past two in the morning and I had just dozed off. I was at the side of him. Just here in this room. I used to sleep on the floor at the side of him. I knew he didn't have long. I was holding his hand. I kissed him good night and said: "I'm going to have a little sleep now, sweetheart." I used to ask him, if he could hear me, to blink his eyes. I said: "Good night, God bless", and I fell asleep. I suddenly woke up and realised I couldn't hear him breathing. Seven weeks I had slept on this floor. I phoned the doctor, and then it was a strange doctor altogether - a locum who came. He stood there and asked "What's the problem then, what's wrong?" I felt like saying: "Well, he's dead, that's the problem".

The doctor said: "No-one told me he was dying or even what kind of a problem there was". I think he meant that he shouldn't have had to come in and ask those questions. He should have had the notes, even if he had been out on his rounds. Somebody should have told him. That was about half past three in the morning and then, the next thing, the police came and that frightened me, because nobody told me they would come.

Harash: Did the doctor inform the police?

Pat: He must have done. I was told later that he had. Well, somebody said it was a matter of course when the coroner had to be informed, but surely, somebody should have told me because it really upset me. I arranged for him to be taken to hospital. I didn't want him being carted away in an ambulance. I wanted it doing respectfully, so I'd arranged for the people who were doing the funeral to bring a special car, but they wouldn't let me stay in the room when they took him away. I was told that it wouldn't be very pleasant after he'd had his autopsy. The death certificate says: "Suspected CJD". The post mortem result confirmed that CJD was the cause of Len's death

Helen Lowe

Helen, age 58, died from CJD in Leeds in 1994. Her daughter, a nurse, and Helen's husband, Colin who cared and looked after her during her 6 months illness describe their frustrations during the course of her illness being investigated. Her daughter at the time, though she was not having the best of relationships with her husband, so perhaps her troubles weren't all in her mind. Helen herself wrote in her diary "They going to test me for mad cow disease." Her symptoms were typical of Narang disease - depression, staggers, falling over and difficulty in walking. They talk to Harash of their experience and the scar it left.

My mother was 58 when she started to become ill in the September of 1993. She began to get headaches and to stagger a bit. These were really bad, blinding headaches she had, migraine type I would say, and she really couldn't cope with them. At about the same time, she seemed to be becoming forgetful. She would ring me up and we'd have a conversation and then she'd ring me back 5 minutes later and have the same conversation again as if she'd forgotten we'd already spoken.

She was having treatment for arthritis and been put on a new medication at that time and I couldn't think of anything else to account for her forgetfulness. Neither of us could think of anything else it could have been. That was the only thing different about her. So, the headaches and the forgetfulness she put down to being side effects. At that time, she was living with her second husband and her son who was 14 at the time.

From September, 1993 to Christmas she had all these staggers and they were getting worse. From about Christmas she felt her speech was slurred and she worried that that, and the way she was staggering, would make people think she was drunk, She didn't drink at all. Her speech was funny, and her walk was funny, she staggered and, every now and again, she jerked and she herself realised it. She lost her balance and when we went shopping she had to hold onto me to keep on a straight line. She wasn't at all keen to see a doctor, and it was only in January, 1994 that a friend of ours, who is a GP, came to visit and thought my mum was quite ill. He got in touch with her GP and she was admitted to hospital in the middle of January. From then until she died just over 2 months later she got worse and worse.

She did fall over a couple of times: she probably staggered and missed her step or something like that. Fortunately, she didn't badly injure herself.

Well, to start right at the beginning of September, she was seeing a Consultant for arthritis. She went there on her own — we didn't know she'd gone —but when she came back, she couldn't remember the name of the Consultant she had seen or what was said and that the consultant wanted her to go in for further investigation. So, I went to the consultant with her and he said that some of her problems weren't related to the arthritis at all. The Consultant couldn't pinpoint exactly what was wrong, and I don't think he really knew what it could be. After all, he was a specialist, a rheumatologist. He couldn't be expected to know everything. He realised something was up and could only advise her having a second opinion. He would like her to go into hospital for investigation

Well, at Christmas time, she was falling asleep time and time again, and sleeping for ages. The other was that she was suffering terrible panic attacks. She started ringing up friends and pouring out her troubles. Whether these were real or imaginary, I don't know. At the time, I though she was not having the best of relationships with her husband, so perhaps her troubles weren't all in her mind. Her husband, though, he certainly thought she was making most of them up. I don't know, but it did make things complicated.

Harash: Right, I know this is one of the big social problems that I have found and it is apparent in some other families.

Her husband and I went with her to the hospital where she was to have all these tests. When we were there, the doctor said that he thought my mother had something seriously wrong.

Well, he made her write her name and he could see her arm twitching and see that she couldn't walk straight. He asked her to count back from 100 in 7s and she could do that perfectly well. She was mentally quite alert and had no problems so far as her memory was concerned..

Her problem was more to do with balancing than with dementia. At that time, she was fully all there. Her brain was all right, even though she sometimes forgot some things. As I said: he did a mental arithmetic thing with her and she knew all the answers. She left him in no doubt about that.

That same day she was admitted to hospital, the doctor said that he would have to start some investigations because, whatever it was, he thought it was quite serious. On the 20th January, she had a lumbar puncture with a blood test and an EEG. On the 21st January, the doctor said that the brain scan had showed something abnormal going on and that he was going to do another scan to find out more the next week. The following day, she had a really bad headaches and a sore neck and, by this time, she was staggering badly on her feet.

Well, you would have thought we would have had the results of these tests straight away but we didn't get the results of these tests at that time."Sorry, we don't have any results on EEG".... "They said nothing showed on EEG". That was the trouble the whole time. I felt we were being fobbed off all the time and, at one point, that I was being led on a wild goose chase. I'm sure he did mention Creutzfeldt Jakob Disease at one point, but when I asked questions, he said that he didn't want to say what it was and didn't want to put words into my mouth. He was looking for something particular, but he wanted me to tell him what it was and, until I did that, he couldn't tell me anything. This went on for weeks on end. One entry in my mother's diary read: "They going to test me for mad cow disease." Obviously, someone had told her so, but who? We could never find out.

This does not tell me much
[illegible] said the doctor instead
of the nurse telling us to see.
They tested me for "mad - cow
disease - result later.

She stayed on in the hospital. The time came when I knew that she was going to die, and I asked about a Hospice, but you can't get someone into a Hospice unless they've only got two weeks to die. In the case of my mum, no-one could predict when she would die: we couldn't move her to a Hospice.

He said that they couldn't know if she had CJD until after she had died. I knew I was being led up the garden path: they threw me a lot of red herrings. I knew that, but I didn't realise you could know so early on. I am a nurse and work in another hospital. Well, because the doctor mentioned CJD, I asked him what it was and how you got. He said: "Oh, we don't know how people get it. It's one of those unfortunate things." I thought about this a lot and, eventually, I did go to the newspapers because I eventually was so exasperated trying to find out about this disease from the hospital people. I went to libraries and things till I felt I had as much information as they had. I felt they just didn't want to tell me anything. Perhaps it was because people have trouble telling people things like that, but I even asked whether my mother was going to die. One doctor said: "Oh, we don't know that." Well, you want to prepare for something like that, but they wouldn't say. This is my opinion. Sometimes it is good to tell people and feel angry that the agony was just being prolonged for reasons of medical procedures.

Well, he must have talked about CJD because, at one point, he did say that, contrary to popular belief and what was in the media, he saw at least 5 to 6 cases a year. That is what he told me. It is strange to find that there is no true figure available of the number suffering this disease and that the only way one can know is by going round to people and asking them in an attempt to find the truth.

The nurses and medical staff didn't seem to give her the normal, close care and attention you might expect while they were handling either my mother. Whether it was because they didn't have the time or for some other reason, I don't know, but she didn't seem to get as much help as might have been given with such things as attending to her teeth and things like that.

She died at around 7 o'clock in the morning. When we went to the hospital, we were told we could go to an office and pick up her things together with a death certificate, but then when we rang up the department to do that, they said: "Oh, I'm sorry, you can't have her death certificate: come back and see the consultant at 5 o'clock". Being myself a nurse, that struck me as rather strange because, if she'd died of CJD, why should we have to come back and see him?

So, we came back at 5 o'clock that afternoon and we had the strangest conversation with the Consultant in his office. He asked us if we were happy with what had happened. I said: "Well, what were they going to put on my mother's death certificate?" The conversation said: "Oh, we'll put CJD on her death certificate, that's no problem." Before she died, there had been hints about dementia, to see where we stood and how we felt about that. I felt that we had been taken in there to see if we would accept dementia and it struck me as very strange that we were being invited back to talk about what was going to go on her death certificate. I asked him what he was going to put on the death certificate and, in the end, he said it would be "CJD". That's what they put on the Certificate so that was OK.

At one, point my mother even suggested to them that she might have this mad cows disease. Mind you, she was a very politically and socially aware woman. She read newspapers, she was very informed and very intelligent. She knew all about this mad cows disease thing anyway from what she had read and seen on the telly, so she was aware of the symptoms and how it affected the animals - and she had been staggering and falling. Whether she meant it or not when she suggested she might have it, I don't know, but she did say it. She had seen some programmes where cows been wobbling. I thought myself she had it when they brought her in from the corridor and her legs went which any way, and she looked just like one of those animals. It was awful really. She looked just like one of those cows you see on the television and I thought: "Well, if they tell me she's not got it, I won't believe them because I could see it". She just looked like they look. I could see it. My mum's brother came from Scotland, and I had to tell him what was going on, so we were all aware of it, watching the symptoms and and how she was behaving. Neither of us are stupid.

It's strange that we spotted what the trouble was, but the doctors either couldn't - or wouldn't. They kept saying they weren't sure and they didn't want to use words which we might repeat. That went on for weeks: it was very strange.

We were told that our permission would be needed if a post-mortem was to be done, but we were also told that that could only be done if someone could be found willing to do it, because it was difficult to find someone prepared to touch her brain. That's what I was told. At any rate, it must have been done almost immediately, because her body was released to the undertaker within a couple of days. They did a post mortem but they didn't tell us the result. She died on the 23rd March 1994.

About the end of February, I think it was, we were asked if a Doctor from Edinburgh could come down to see us because, at that point, my mother's sister had died. She had similar symptoms in a way but, as it happens, she'd had a blood clot on her brain. We were in with him for probably 2 hours. He asked us lots of questions, what my mother ate and all about her life style and her family history. I asked him how she got it and he admitted that he didn't know, but was positive that you couldn't get it from eating meat, blah, blah, blah. So, why was he so interested in asking what she ate, I wanted to know? He said it was for research. That was the end of that, but, when somebody asks whether your mother ate eye balls and things like that, you wonder why. Another thing the Doctor from Edinburgh said was that there was a 10% chance that it would be passed on as a hereditary thing and that worried me because I have daughters. He didn't tell me whether or not I should have tests but just insisted that it was not a disease you could catch from anything.

It was only when she was in her 30s that she came down from Scotland to Leeds with her second husband. She had been born in Stirling and we lived in Scotland till we came South. At home, we tended to eat stews and mince because they were cheap and we never ate pork till we came to England. We had mince and potatoes as a Scottish dish and steak pie. Chicken was only for special occasions. I remember my grandmother was a great one for soup with a big piece of mutton in it.

She just used to get a big piece of mutton, my grandma, and boil it for a couple of hours. It wasn't the brain she used, just the meat of sheep. Boiled beef, she called it, but ,because beef would be more expensive, it was mutton she used, definitely.

She'd boil that for a couple of hours with vegetables, lentils and things like that to make soup.

When she was younger and living in Scotland, she did suffer from psoriasis, quite badly sometimes, and regularly went to hospital in Glasgow twice a week for treatment. It would flare up if she got stressed or was upset. She had it quite badly. She had it on her elbows and on her face, her back and her legs. Sunlight helped it but she never really got rid of it: it was always there.

She didn't have any pets, she hated cats. My father, he worked on a farm when he was young, he was a country sort of boy, and then he was a lorry driver when we were children.

Colin 2nd Husband talks to Harash

We had been married for about 19 years when Helen's trouble began at the end of the 1993 summer, in about September. She had arthritis and that was a big problem which probably hid the start of what was to follow. A lot we just wrote off as side effects from the medications she was taking and were continually being changed. She had a good memory, but she did start that summer to be forgetful on the odd time or two. She would go shopping and forget to bring something she needed. That was unlike her, she never used to forget anything. By about September or October, I was noticing it and beginning to say: "Oh, well, your memory is getting as bad as mine now." That is when we thought, "Yes there were changes in Helen".

Her balance problems started about October. To begin with, we really thought it was only the side effects of the drugs she was taking for arthritis. She'd changed her medication in September and we knew that the side effects were common. During the night, when she'd get up to go to the toilet, or something like that, she'd say: "Oh, I feel dizzy." It was just a momentary thing, you know, it wasn't any prolonged thing but it went on for 2 or 3 weeks

She was seeing the doctor regularly with her arthritis and the doctor found that she had an ear infection, so she was given treatment for that, so, we then decided it was side effects from the infected ear and not from the arthritis. We just assumed that was it. We dismissed the arthritis side effects and thought it was the infected ear.

By the beginning of December, she could not balance herself. She really had a bad time. She'd changed medication constantly and each time she'd had bad side effects. She said to me: "I don't want any more medication for a few weeks. I want to clear all these out of my system." She physically was looking bad and was starting to look drawn.

Over Christmas and the New Year we thought: "Oh well, she'll start to feel better soon, but she'll get the arthritis pain back", but she didn't seem to get the arthritis pain back and she never mentioned it.

She showed no signs of getting better whatever, so that took us straight into January when she had her first dip. So that's how I see it, living there all the time. I mean, sometimes I think I was too close to her.

I'd go out at quarter past seven and she'd get up after me and get Stuart up to get off to school. He's 14. On the 11th January, I got up and woke Stuart and, although Helen wasn't well, I had to leave her and go off to work. At 10 o'clock, I got a phone call from our friend Daniel, who had called in for a chat and a coffee, but was so concerned that he rang her GP. The GP came down and his first thought was that she'd a blood clot or something, her behaviour was so far from normal. He rang me up and I came home and it was rather confusing at that point. She was walking about and her GP was arranging for a neurologist to come up and see her next day. Actually, at quarter past seven that morning, when I had left, you could see her confusion, she was asking the same question, again and again. Certainly, she was not normal.

Nothing happened during that week. I kept making a lot of phone calls to see what was happening. Every time I rang the hospital, I was put through to a Secretary and she didn't know anything about it. By Friday, I managed to get through to a neurologist and was told they would give her a brain scan.

I understand that they did two EEGs and various scans. On the first day she went for the brain scan, Tuesday, they took her down to St. James Hospital. Now, at that time, I'd been at home with her, all the time, for seven days. it was like full time nursing in a way, because she was so confused you couldn't really leave her because, if you did, like you say, she'd turn the gas on or something like that. For seven days, she never knew what day it was. At that point I knew there was something seriously wrong with her. That's why I'd taken her along for an appointment. I'd had seven days of it. There was something seriously wrong and I just couldn't cope.

I couldn't go on like this and I wanted her in hospital and, when we went to the hospital I thought it would to come to a row if they wouldn't admit her,because I was not going out of there with her and taking her home. She sat down in front of the doctor and he said: "What day is it." She said: "Tuesday." He says what's the date and she says: "the 18th January, 1994". I couldn't believe it. I thought that was quite remarkable. She was answering every question perfectly, a think she' hadn't done for several days. The doctor said: "I want you to count down now in 7s from 100." So she started counting down and he said: "Wait a minute." He couldn't write them down fast enough, she was just rattling them off like that. I just couldn't believe it. We took her through into another room, where there was this rheumatologist person. At that point, all we knew was she had this rheumatology problem and then, at the end of examination, he said: "We need to keep her in, but we haven't got any of the right beds available. We'll keep her in a bed somewhere for the time being, and then later transfer her to neurology."

Her staggering and unsteadiness on her feet, which had been very noticeable when she was at home, got worse from the time she went into hospital. Her walk got to the point where I used to call it like a jig, you know, because she used to go like zig zag pattern. We used to make a joke of it. Coming into the ward, we were all doing that little jig to imitate her. It didn't go on long like that, because, soon, she couldn't walk on her own. Within a couple of weeks she was in a wheel chair. She couldn't even make the toilet. You had to go with her because she couldn't control her hand and be able to make it do what she wanted.

When she was sitting and she went to pick up a glass or cup, she had to watch her hand where it was going. She couldn't do it automatically, you know, like you change the gears in your car, she couldn't do that. We bought her a twin handled cup, but it wasn't very long before she couldn't control that either. She could get two hands on it, one on each side, but even then it was her co-ordination that was going all the time.

You see, she had this confusion, but every now and again, between bouts of confusion there would be absolute clarity. In my mind, I was sure it was the medication for the arthritis which was at the back of it all. I was not linking mad cows disease with Helen at that stage, although Helen had written that in her book earlier on.

The trouble was, I was being told nothing. I was going in every night, but nobody was speaking to me. All they would tell me when I'd get to the nursing station was, "Well, this is what's happened today you know".....”Oh she's had this test and they couldn't pin anything down." I never saw a doctor,only the nurses and I knew they couldn't tell me anything, because they obviously didn't know anything. At the same time nobody was talking to me and that went on for five weeks.

I thought : "I'm her husband and everybody keeps saying nobody knows what's wrong with her. Surely, they should be asking me about her, how she had got on at home, what she had been like. After all, I had been living with her for 24 hours a day." I took some time off with Stuart and we went down and on the Friday night and the Sunday afternoon. Both sets of staff had said the best time to come was at 1 o'clock when Mr. B starts. I went on Monday at 1 o'clock and he was on holiday. I was really annoyed at that because I had spoken to two lots of nursing staff and been told that he was coming on Monday. I wanted to see a doctor, because nobody was talking to me, nobody was telling me anything.

At the end, I did see the Registrar but all he would say to me was that he really didn't know. I'd be better to see Mr. B, who was dealing with it. He sent the Secretary to make an appointment and the appointment was for 10 days later. So Helen was in 6 or 7 weeks before I saw Mr. B for a second time and he seemed surprised that I should want to see him. He said he couldn't really help me. At some point during that meeting, "Jacob" was mentioned. Most other things had been eliminated by then, he said: so they were really left with nothing much else.....

The one thing which always sticks in my mind, and this was just a week or two before she died actually,was that one night, when the nurses were turning her in her bed, I noticed Helen had this absolute stark terror on her face. Now years ago, Helen and I used to follow the mad cow thing....I remember seeing cattle, seeing their eyes, that's what sticks in my memory, and I saw that same look in Helen's eyes that night. I'd never seen her like that before that night when the nurses were turning her. It was the same look as I had seen on the cows on the telly. I didn't get that idea because I had been thinking about mad cows disease and linking it in any way with Helen. It was when they were handling her in the bed, it flashed into my mind from the expression on her face. It was the expression and the sheer stark terror in her face and her eyes. I couldn't believe it and instantly the picture of the mad cows came up in my mind. Helen's face was sort of like a mad cow.

Yes, I know what Helen had written in her diary right at the beginning of her being in hospital, and before anybody was thinking in terms of mad cows disease, but that isn't what made me think it. It was the look in her face. A lot of people have since said to me that she did know that she had mad cow disease, but I always argued that she did not know what she had, even though she had written it herself: "mad cows disease, get the results later". But, at that stage, nobody was talking about mad cows disease. Nobody was mentioning it whatsoever at that time. It was never mentioned. It did not come up. They were looking at Alzheimer and I was thinking of Alzheimer and that was what was in my mind. After Helen had been ill for two or three weeks, I was wondering how I would handle the rest of my life full time with her, twenty four hour day, if she came out of hospital in the state she was in. I was worried, though that's a dreadful thing to have to admit but it could go on for years if it was Alzheimer. Nobody was thinking in terms of BSE, mad cow CJD was not mentioned. She knew all about mad cow disease and had followed its development from the TV. Helen was very volatile and excitable and could get really worked up about things and this mad cow thing was one of the things which had excited her. That entry in the diary was really a self-diagnosis.

She didn't say much about the visitors she'd had, but people would read her diary which, to begin with, she was writing every day and they would write in it too because, if they didn't, after they'd gone, she would forget that they had been. She'd look in the diary and she say: "Oh, so-and-so been." It would remind her. She did this with everything, not just friends and relatives, anybody. Whoever actually visited her wrote in the diary, it's in the diary. She could keep reading it to know who had come. She could be quite alert and with-it from time to time. Once I was standing beside the bed with this nurse and I had it in my mind that the medicine had to do with the condition she was in. I was talking to the nurse and I said: "Surely, it can't be the medication she was on from September to December that caused all this", and the nurse said: "Well, what was she on?" Helen was sitting there listening and Helen said: "I'm on such and such a thing." So she knew what she was on, and she was hearing the conversation, even though there was a lot of confusion. The nurse said: "Oh well, you need an awful lot of that to cause any kind of problems you know." Helen then immediately said "Oh well, wait a minute, each human being is different." Now, in spite of all the confusion, there was an absolute flash of logic. The nurses were aware of the diary, although I don't think anybody in the hospital paid particular attention to it other than the visitors.

She had been intrigued, almost fascinated, by mad cows disease and I just thought it was something from her sub-conscious which has come out and she'd related to it. Before she took ill, when it came on the news, she used to sit in that chair and she'd get quite worked up about it saying: "It's a cover up", but then that's the kind of person she was on that subject. In the ward, when I told Ivy, who was in a bed across from her all the time Helen was in the ward, what she had died from, Ivy had no doubts. "Oh well", she claimed: "Helen always did say she had that, you know." She must have mentioned it to the other patients in the ward, and, probably also, to the nurses.

Harash: Now, if she mentioned that they had tested her for this "mad cows" disease, did she ever mention what the results were. Did she ever get the results? Were you ever told? She just wrote that in the diary. That's Helen's writing.

Yes, well that was a week after she went in, the Tuesday after

Helen had written that reference to Mad Cow Disease, they were going to do another EEG, were just waiting for an appointment. So, she was saying they were looking for CJD as early as that. We were getting nothing back from them, all they were saying was that they were testing. Oh, yes, it was quite a while on before it was suggested that they were left with nothing else. These EEG tests were done twice.

Harash: When you were talking to this Consultant about the death certificate, can you remember anything he said while you were with him. You did say you had a long one hour chat.

I had the feeling that he was probing to find out our views on the mad cows disease. At the end of the day, you know, if it was proved that Jacobs and mad cows were linked together, it would in a way be a big problem for the Government in handling the situation on beef. I felt as though he was seeing how we would handle it and I thought he was mainly interested in whether we were going to go to the press. We had another case of mad cows disease in Leeds you see. You have to learn to treat it very very carefully.

He just talked generally for an hour round the whole subject of Helen's death in a way. To me as I said, he was probing how I was going to feel. He was going to put CJD on her Death Certificate but I think he felt that it might appear in the local press that a woman had died in St. James from mad cows disease and for that reason, was uncomfortable. I'd a feeling that something else was going to be on the death certificate. The whole gist, why did it take an hour for him to eventually give us the death certificate and why didn't he have it with him in that room. We had to go down a corridor and he disappeared. I thought that he went out and actually wrote the death certificate. I don't know, maybe I've got it wrong there, but he had to go and get it and I thought he's gone to make it out.

You asked what we used to eat. Well, we didn't eat mince much. I don't know what you've heard. You've probably been told we ate a lot of mince because that appeared in this big banner headline. We ate a lot of beef and a lot of steaks but not many burgers. We rarely ate them. Occasionally she would bring mince pies home from the bakers shop, the little Scotch things. She had all those kind of jobs. She did eat a lot of meat in her previous marriage.

Well, the things I remember, which we miss now, because I'm having to learn to cook. Potato and leek soup was a regular, because she could make that. We went off beef at one stage until Stuart and I protested that we didn't want to be vegetarians, so the beef reappeared. Unfortunately, you hear one thing one day from the experts and the opposite the next day and it seems to turn upside down.

She worked in a hotel for a few weeks, cooking. She had some office jobs until Stuart was born and then, when Stuart was two year old, she went back part time to Sainsburys.

Harash: Could you tell me condition of her teeth?

Teeth, oh, excellent, only once did she have a filling.

Harash: Now do you have any questions to ask me while I'm here?

Not off hand, probably when you've gone it'll all start coming back and I'll think why didn't I ask this, and why didn't I ask that. I am not worried about myself, but tell me what chance there is of Stuart has developing CJD. Could it be hereditary?

Harash: I do not believe that it is truly hereditary, because it's caused by a virus. It's not in the genes.

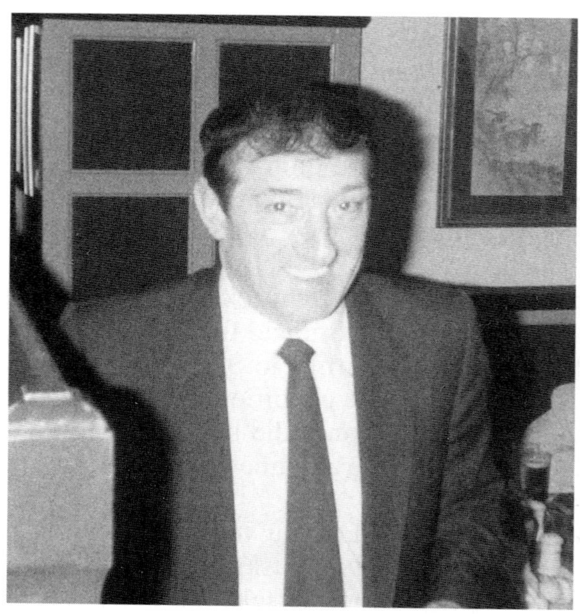

Ralph Boutflower

Ralph Boutflower, a keen meat-eater, died in 1989. The first sign of trouble was when Ralph, from Sunderland, complained about problems with his eyes. He became frightened, and the fear grew so intense that he could not put one foot in front of the other. He forgot who his children were. Ralph, who had worked as a steel milling machinist, was born and grew up in the East End of London. He had a taste for frying up thick beefburgers. His wife, Sarah, 57, describes how the disease killed him at the age of 53. We did not have a potst-mortem, but then it was a coincidence that when Ralph was in Newcastle General Hospital, a brain biopsy was done. By my his touch method, I had confirmed he had CJD. Sarah describes how she and her children only realised the connection with BSE when pictures of cows collapsing with the disease appeared on television. Her son said to her: "That's exactly how my dad went."

We celebrated our 25th wedding anniversary on 28th March 1989. There wasn't anything wrong, nothing at all wrong with Ralph. My birthday was on 29th April and we enjoyed ourselves. He was completely normal, just the way he always was and it wasn't until the first week in May that he started complaining about his eyes.

Ralph was tiling the bathroom in May 1989 when, for the first time, he complained to me about his eyes. He kept rinsing them with cold water. He was unable to see to the side of his eyes. I thought it was because he was working in a confined space, so I asked him to leave it alone, but he insisted on finishing it. We went to the doctor's, and they said it was vertigo and gave him treatment for that. Ralph found it easier if he wore dark glasses.

Then the weight started dropping off him and he started losing all co-ordination, falling about and everything. From that time he just went downhill very quickly.

Whenever anybody came in to the room, he would jump. He would not be aware initially when someone came in, but, as the person passed in front of him, into his field of vision, he would jump and be terrified.

He became increasingly frightened: you could see the fear on his face. When our son, a nurse, returned from a late shift, his dad would try to work his way into the back of the settee, terrified of him. One day, I brought in some washing, and there was a greenfly on my hand. I said: "Look at the greenfly." He looked at it and jumped back, saying: "That's not a greenfly. It's too big." He was frightened of it. The least little thing was frightening him. It became so bad that he could not put one foot in front of the other. He used to creep about the floor because he felt safer doing that than walking.

He would sit and stare at the television, and I would say: "Put the television on if you want." He would crawl across, but he did not know what to press, and I would say: "I'll put it on for you." He stared at the television without knowing what was on. If there was a play on, he would not be able to follow it. Sometimes, he would roll his thumbs while sitting.

Through the night, he would talk in his sleep. He would talk about the cows in the meadow. Then he would be adding up: "22 and 30 - I can't remember what that makes", I would hear him say. I would wake him. "You're talking in your sleep Ralph," I would say. He would reply: "I do not know what you mean. Have I been talking again?" And then he would sit up in bed. He would say: "I do not know what is the matter with me."

He had sudden jerks over his whole body. He would move his legs suddenly during the night. His legs would jerk, and he would sit up, and then lie back down. I never told him to stop because I knew he was not doing it deliberately. I knew that there was something wrong. Then the weight started dropping off him and he was becoming forgetful and confused. If he heard a song on the radio that reminded him of a chalet holiday we had had, he would ask: "Are we in the chalet?" That was when I started realising that there was something drastically wrong. If he had to go to a specific place, he would want me to go with him. He thought that he might either catch the wrong bus, or not find the place where he was supposed to go.

He would be fascinated about what was behind closed doors, and would ask whether he could see what was behind them. I would say: "You can, it's your house, do what you like." He would open the door, and act as though he was like a little boy in a toy shop. It was as if everything was strange to him. He could not recognise a thing.

He lost all co-ordination; he was falling about. He could not feed himself, he would miss his mouth. We had to feed him, or he would say: "I'm not hungry," so that he would not have to feed himself. At times, he would talk gibberish, saying things that had no meaning. He would start off talking sensibly, and go on to something that had nothing to do with what he had been saying. I would say: "I don't know what you're talking about Ralph." His speech was not slurred. It was his mind that must have been all jumbled up.

At the end of May, he forgot who we were. He did not know his two sons or his daughter. He did not know who anybody was. He just forgot everything, although he could remember events from when he was a little boy ,but eventually, his long-term memory went as well.

From the start of his taking bad, he became steadily worse very quickly over ten weeks. Our 25th wedding anniversary was on March 28th, and my 50th birthday was on April 29th, and there was nothing wrong with him at all at that time. He was just normal.

In September, he saw a neurologist. I had thought he would not still be with us by then, the way he was going and that doctor immediately said that he wanted Ralph admitted for tests. Ralph was so scared and nervous.

In hospital, his eyes were just stary; he just stared looking vacantly into space, there was nothing behind them. Our son said: "Close your eyes dad." But he did not know how to close his eyes. Our son said: "I'll have to close my dad's eyes because they will be dry." He closed Ralph's eyes, and he never opened them again for the three weeks he was in hospital. They asked me to try to get him to drink water because he was dehydrating, but he would not open his mouth for them. I would say: "Open your mouth, Ralph." I would pull his chin down, and squirt in the water. I would shut his mouth, and say: "Now swallow," and he would swallow it. He did not even know how to chew.

They would put meals down for him, but he could not eat them. If I was there, I would feed him. I would give him a drink, but he would spit it out. He did not know how to pick the knife and fork up.

They gave him a lumbar puncture and brain scans. They had to sedate him to do the lumbar puncture. A young lady doctor who did it did say that he had all the symptoms of CJD. They had had a case in just before him with exactly the same symptoms.

They asked us to go in on the Tuesday. They were talking about taking a bit of his brain away to test, a biopsy, and after that had been done they told us that he had CJD, and that there was no cure, no treatment, nothing they could do to help him. He was just asleep all the time. He stayed there in the hospital for three weeks, until he died.

They were positive it was CJD. Even when he died, they did not have a post-mortem because they said they knew what it was. They asked to have a post-mortem but I refused. It was something he had not wanted to happen to him, so I said: "No". They said: "We know what he has died of, so we can fill the certificate in." They put CJD on his death certificate. They said that if the coroner wanted a post-mortem, they would have had to do one. I know now he should have had a post-mortem. There is a lot of cover-up. The Government just does not want to know about it.

By the time he died, he just looked like a skeleton. He must have been about six stone. He had been 12 stone. When he was lying in the bed, you could count every rib, every bone in his body.

Ralph was a meat fan. He ate all kinds of meat. He had lots of liver. He loved meat pies. He would eat ox tail, or pig's head. He would boil a pig's head and make a soup out of it and, when he was a boy, his mother had often bought sheep's heads and made soup out of them. It was the way of life then in the East End, although I do not think Ralph himself bought sheep's head.

When he was a little boy, his cousin used to take him to a farm for a holiday at Hornsby, a couple of hours away. We used to have a cat and a dog. He used to buy meat from the butcher's for the dog during the 1980s. **He went one day and the butcher said: "I have got it but we are waiting for someone to come and test it."** He used to boil it all up in a separate pan, what we called dog's pan.

He used to go to the market in Newcastle to buy thick beef-burgers, and come home and fry them with onions. He used to eat loads of them. I myself did not eat red meat. He used to eat the weirdest things, would try everything. He used to say: "There's no good saying you don't like something until you've tried it." He thoroughly enjoyed his food, and he used to like preparing it. He was made redundant as a steel milling machinist in 1980, and after he finished work he prepared everything.

The children used to eat a little bit beef, but not much. I have a daughter and two sons, one of them married with two children. Now, they do not eat beef at all after the way their dad went. They say that there must be a link with meat. Ralph had not had injections of the growth hormone, which I am told has also caused CJD.

When we saw those BSE cows on television falling over, we could see that it was the same as what had hit Ralph. He was unable to keep his balance in just the same way as the cows. My son, who was a nurse, first noticed it. He pointed to a cow falling over on television and said: "Look at that. Just what does not remind you of?" It reminded us all of Ralph. He said that there had to be a connection. "That's what it was," he said. "That's exactly how my dad went."

Harash: What about his teeth, did he any problems with his teeth at all?

He had full dentures fitted in 1980 and, before that, he had dentures at the front, the two front ones. Those he got before we were married and he had them for years and years. When his other teeth started to decay the dentist decided to take the lot out and make him a whole set.

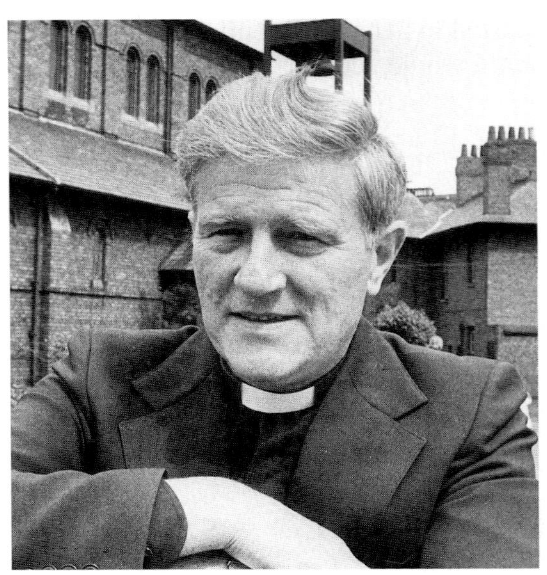

Kevin Stock

Kevin, an active parish priest, of St Columbus Church, Sunderland died at the age of 63 in 1993 after being diagnosed as suffering from CJD. His symptoms started with balancing and shaking similar to those seen in BSE cattle typical of Narang disease. His sister, Brenda Gilbert describes how these clinical symptoms progressed while her brother was still busy collecting funds for changing of church bell which he wanted to complete before he died.

I first became aware that there was something amiss with Kevin when he took some people to Birmingham airport and lost his way. After all that was a run he had done it hundreds of times. He could not find the way, just did not know which way to turn. It was then I realised he was ill. I took the car keys away from him. How he avoided having accidents I don't know.

It was about six weeks before that that I went from Birmingham to Somerset with him. At that time, his reactions were quite good because when a swan flew down in front of the car and he had to break, he did so instantly and without any difficulty. From time to time, he seemed to have to explain things to people over and over again as though he thought they weren't understanding him. We went to get a rail card for him at a railway station and he had to keep asking how he could use it. He had to keep on repeating it over and over again.

My mother is 93 now and at that time had some problems on her old property. I went with Kevin to get a new roof done, and he was almost embarrassingly loud, talking to the contractors who were doing the job. He kept on and on. I ended up saying: "Ken they must know what to do, so you don't have to keep saying it again and again." He was not that sort of person who normally repeated himself. He could converse with Bishops, Lords, and anyone else. He didn't have a problem like that.

He was still the parish priest when he died. Although he had made up his mind to retire he was still an active priest.

The first time I knew he was seriously ill was when I phoned to see whether he would be able to come to my 60th birthday celebration. When I got off the phone, I said to my husband, "Either Ken is drunk, or there is something the matter with him. I can't understand anything he is saying." So I phoned David Smith, a friend, because I knew that he was in reasonably frequent touch with my brother. He said: "I don't know what is the matter with him, but there is something terribly wrong with him."

I phoned up some parishioners of his parish and they said: "Oh, thank goodness you phoned us, we didn't know your surname. We were at our wits end to know what to do, we know he is ill." We went to see him and he obviously was ill. He could not concentrate on anything. He was emotional, and we went to see his doctor, and he thought he might have a brain tumour and would arrange for tests.

What Ken was saying didn't relate to anything, just had no bearing on what I was talking about. But it wasn't slurred speech. It just didn't make any sense. He was agitated really. He was upset that he couldn't remember what he wanted to remember as well as he had normally done.

Every now and again, when he walked, he lurched. I just remember he would be walking along and suddenly he would be down and he would pick himself up again. In the house it would be always to the right side, I think, because he would go down the passage but whether that was because the wall was there and it was convenient to support himself on that wall but he always supported himself all down the passage against the wall. I went out with him in the evening on his own, and he seemed to get better when he was out on his own with just me walking down the road. He slept a lot as well, and he would sit in a chair and sleep very fitfully and then he would wake, but I think at night he didn't sleep very well at all. It would have been September, October of 1991. His condition was changing very quickly.

Only a few weeks before, that during that summer when they were going to change the hanging of the bells, he had raised £30,000 for the fund, mostly on his own. By September and October he was too ill. Half way through a service he, would forget the words and that is after 40 years of knowing them.

He seemed to be very worked up about it, but then he was a perfectionist and as usual he was very keyed up wanting everything to be perfect. I was not aware there was anything seriously wrong with him. How much his illness contributed to his agitation, at that time, I am not sure. When he was sitting down he would twitch. He was twitching when he was asleep, and that would be 1991 November, December.

His twitching became much more erratic. His hands would twitch a lot, and so would his legs. I cannot say whether it was one leg or both legs. He would even jump. The thing that upset him was he would be half way through a sentence and he couldn't finish it, because he couldn't think what else to say. Writing a letter, he couldn't do it.

Harash: Did he complain of anything being wrong with him?

One of his parishioners has told me that he did complain about pains in his legs, that his balance was bad, his memory was failing, he was unable to settle, he was very emotional and he could read or concentrate to finish what he was doing. The thing that sticks in my mind is the lady whose wedding we're going to on Sunday. He said to her, "Elspeth, my brain feels like a sponge". He actually said my brain feels like a sponge. He said he had pain in his legs and he did not seem to be able to get comfortable. He kept moving from one place to another.

His eyesight had really deteriorated when we went to see him in Neurological Centre in Sunderland. By then, he didn't know us. He got even our names all muddled. He put the wrong surnames to Christian names. He knew we were related in some way, although at times he just couldn't sort people out, know who was who. Then he would have a sudden burst of recovery, because he remembered who Sarah was, that's our daughter, and she had just had the baby and we had a card from her and he was amused by that. It was a very amusing card. He was losing a lot of weight at that stage. We live in Essex, but we tried to make certain that there was somebody with him all the time.

To begin with he was a very sensible man. I think the thing that struck us was the change in personality and mood which was our greatest worry. The first real test that was done was a brain scan, a CAT scan. That was after we had been to see the doctor. He thought it probably was a tumour. The scan showed negative. We all thought it means, "Oh, he hasn't got a brain tumour at all." We all had a drink, and celebrated.

After he had been only a few days in the Neurological Centre, the doctor, for the first time, told us straight out what the trouble was. Well, he said: "It is the human equivalent of mad cow disease." He did not use the words CJD. That was in 1991 and Kevin died in August 1992. Yes, we were told: "It was a form of mad cow disease." The first time I saw him in hospital was just before Christmas we saw him, and from then on he was worse every time we went to see him. He had difficulty in explaining. He didn't answer. He just progressively got worst.

He had several operations on his throat. He was very very afraid of needles and, therefore, never volunteered as blood donor.

Harash: What about his teeth.

I honestly don't know how many fillings he had. He certainly had fillings but he did not have dentures. Strangely, because he was ill I had to cancel dentist's visits he was due to make.

He used to go to Birmingham market. And, I think when he had these evenings, he would go to market then. He used to bulk buy, yes. He didn't have a lot of commercial food. He wasn't a frozen food man at all. He enjoyed cooking and he would cook his food from fresh, and it might well be that he had cheap meat because he didn't earn very much so he didn't buy expensive cuts of meat.

Harash: I know that he used to work and help cooking food in some pub.

He actually served in one of the pubs up here. When he went to his new parish there was a pub opposite. They were short staffed once and he said: "Well I've done a bit of bar work and cooking. I'll come in and help out at lunch times." He was a very good cook and he used to do an English night or Greek night or something to raise funds for the church. He was certainly cooking up until he became seriously ill. He would make brawn. He would do it from a pig's head, ox tail and bones and things for the soups. There were butchers in his congregation and they would say: "Here's a bone for soup".

He often did have nicks and scratches because he always fooling about with the dog. He would be playing with lumps of wood on the beach with the dog, then throw them for the dog to pull it and he would certainly would have cuts and scratches on his hands. One clergy house he had for a while backed on to a farm and he often used to go and feed the cows sugar lumps.

Peter Hall also died of CJD while a student at Monk Wearmouth College, right at the back of my brothers church.

Barbara Lydiatt

Barbara Lydiatt died from CJD in January, 1993 at the age of 37, four months after the initial symptoms of the disease appeared. A year before her death, she had moved home to live nearer to her sisters. Her symptoms started with depression, balancing and shaking, similar to those seen in BSE cattle, and typical of Narang disease. She had four children, then aged between 14 and 21, and had separated from her husband. Her sister's experiences with the medical staff left her infuriated. A year after Barbara's death, Cindy tells Harash Narang how the disease took her sister from complete health to death in four months. She did have a link with Ashford, Kent where she lived in a farm cottage and helped with cattle on the farm.

On June 12th 1992, we went out to celebrate her 37th birthday. Barbara was fine then. The next month we went out dancing on the flat roof of the public house around the corner trying to raise money for the Telethon, Children in Need. We were in fancy-dress clothes, and we danced on the roof for four hours to attract attention and raise money for charity. We walked the streets in fancy-dress with collection buckets to raise money for the Telethon. She was certainly fine and full of life then.

Our mum had leukemia, and died at the age of 39. Her mum (our grandmother) died about 17 years ago at a ripe old age, and her sister is still alive. My mum's sister still lives in Kennington, about two miles from Ashford, Kent, in the same house where my mum was brought up.

My sister Barbara, we called her Bamsy, lived on a farm when she was 18. It was a tied farm cottage where she lived for about four years. Her husband was a lorry driver, and they had the cottage adjoining the farmer's house. If help was needed with the farm, her husband was supposed to help. He used to be a long distance lorry driver and, when he was away on a trip, which he was most of the time, my sister used to end up helping the farmer. She used to feed the animals. I can remember because once when I was over staying with her, she actually helped a calf being born in the early hours of one morning.

It was September 1992 when things started to go wrong. Suddenly, for no reason, she fell down the stairs. Within a couple of days, she said she had pains in her back and shoulder, so I took her to the doctor's. He sent her for an X-ray, and were told that there was nothing wrong. Then she developed an awful cough, a really bad cough. I took her back to the doctor's. He examined her chest and said it was fine. Then she developed a rash all over her body, a bit like a heat rash, tiny spots on the skin. I took her back to the doctor's. He just said it could be due to the heat.

Next, she started falling over. She started staggering around as though she was drunk, falling from side to side, usually to the left hand-side. Her left hand was shaking. It was not just a little shake, it was jerking continuously. She would fall into fences, slumping forward. She would have no control over her balance; she could not walk straight. I was extremely worried about her and took her to the doctor's. The doctor told me she had a nervous breakdown, which I could not credit as she was so happy being down here with her twin sisters. He did not prescribe her anything. He merely said there was nothing they could do.

We brought her home. We were trying to care for her, hoping to build her confidence up and that she would get better. She did not get any better, she became worse. She repeated herself, asking the same question over again, forgetting what she had been told. She would sit and shut one eye to look at you. I would say: "Why are you doing that?" and she would say: "I can't see you, you are all blurred. If I shut one eye, I can see you better."

She lived across the road from us. We would regularly look in to see if she was all right, but she usually preferred not to get out of bed. Previously, she used to spend quite a bit of time with us, and I was trying my best to encourage her to get out of bed and come across to us, but she would not do that any more. One day I went over and she had wet the bed. She had a go at me that day because I told the doctor, and she was so embarrassed. I said: "It's important, I must tell the doctor." We took her to the doctor's at least 3 times but all we were told was that she'd had a breakdown and there was nothing they could do.

The time came when I tried to get her up, but her legs just would not hold her body weight. I phoned the doctor's, but they refused to come to see her. Once again, they said she had a breakdown and there was nothing they could do. I rang my local hospital, crying and told them the doctor would not come out. She was shaking rapidly. She could not stand up. She was wetting the bed, and I could not cope any more. They said they would ring the doctor and tell him to come out.

The doctor came out and said: "There's nothing I can do for her." Me and my twin sister said: "Well, you sit there. She can't be left on her own. You sit and look after her, we are going." We weren't really going to go, but we were hoping he'd take her in hospital and find out what was wrong and we walked out the door. He did nothing, packed his briefcase and left. I really wanted him to take her into hospital.

We ran back into the house and I was crying and I phoned the hospital and said: "I am bringing her up." We borrowed the money, put her in a taxi and took her to the hospital. They had a psychiatrist to see her. I said: "We are not taking her home. We've got to find out what is wrong with her?"

She was swearing really terribly. We are not a coarse or foul-mouthed family, but she was saying some really terrible swear-words, which was most unlike her - especially in a public place.

A psychiatrist came, and said: "I don't know what it is, but it's certainly not a mental problem." They put her into a ward in the hospital. I can remember trying to come out of the ward, and she was shouting: "Cindy, Cindy."

They said: "Can you please tell her to be quiet." I told her, "You've got be quiet, I've got to go now." This was in the early hours of the morning. As soon as I went to walk away, "Cindy" she shouted. They said she woke up the whole ward.

They did numerous tests on her. They did a lumbar puncture and I was told that this came back, 'high in protein on the brain'. They moved her to another hospital for further tests. By this time, she was totally immobile. She had to be picked up and put in a wheelchair to be moved around.

We haven't got a mum or a dad, they're both dead. I was known as her next of kin. I rang and asked to see a consultant, and a lady doctor took me into a side ward and said: "We've tested her for everything that we can, and its all come back negative. She is showing signs of a rare virus." I said: "What is it?

The doctor said: "It's Creutzfeldt-Jakob Disease. She is showing the signs of it. There is no test that proves she has it, but she is showing the signs. I asked: "What are you telling me?"

She said: "If she has the virus there's nothing we can do. We cannot stop it, and if we could, we can't repair the damage it's already caused and, with the rapid deterioration she is showing, she will not last years."

"Are you telling me my sister's going to die now? Just tell me what's going on," and she just put her head down.

I was in an awful state. I could not believe what I was hearing. I did not want to ask any more questions, but I could not believe what I was being told. I had never heard the words she used before. In fact, when I got back to my twin, I could not remember the words she had said. All I could remember was that I was told that she was showing signs of a virus. My twin asked: "What she's got?" I said: "I don't know."

She was transferred back because there was nothing more they could do for her, and it would be easier for her to be nearer us. It was on her medical records that she had CJD. The consultant said that the only positive test that could prove it 100 per cent was a brain biopsy. Six other consultants had seen my sister, and in their opinion they were 90 per cent certain she had CJD. If I wanted the test, they would do it. I said: "If I let you do the test, is there anything you can do to save my sister?" They said: "No, it will only confirm what I'm saying." I said: "You're not going to cut her head open. She's gone through enough already."

By this time, she was incontinent. It used to embarrass her. She was totally immobile: she could not even hold her head up. Her speech was extremely slurred. She complained that she could hardly see us, we were just a blur all the time.

She was calmer when she was lying down. Her legs used to shake, but the shaking was worst in her hands. It seemed to settle more when she was lying down. If you tried to sit her up, and put her into a wheelchair, she shook worse. She complained continuously if you tried to brush her hair. She would say: "Please don't brush my hair, my head hurts." She cried so much, and she never used to cry.

She used to get excited when you cuddled her. She loved a cuddle. If you cuddled her, she used to laugh. She would laugh a lot, and she would start shaking as she laughed.

She was put on an open ward, but the nurses were so short-staffed that my sister was not being cared for in the way she needed. She was extremely frightened, she did not know what was going on. She kept shouting out: "Get me out of bed. Take me for a cigarette." She could not do anything for herself, she relied on other people. I spent as much time as I could at the hospital with her, but one day I went up there, they were so short-staffed that the day nurses had left her in her bed. She was all dirty. She'd got sores on her where she'd been laying three hours dirty and when I saw that, I said: "I'm taking her out of this hospital. I'm using your hoist to bath her because she had to be hoisted. There was nothing I could do but take her home. I just said: "I'm taking her out of this place."

That was January 2nd. My GP told me not to bring her home because I would be unable to cope. There would be convulsions, coma, and so on. I was told all this but I could not see my sister all dirty in the hospital with no-one to care for her. I still thought I could care for her better at home rather than keep spending all my time at the hospital and trying to find people to look after my children while I was there.

I asked for an ambulance to take her home, but they said I could not have one due to cut-backs. I would have to book one hours in advance. So I bathed her, dried her hair, and had her daughter come up in a car. I asked for some nappies or anything like that but they said I couldn't have any. I just took them: I took them because I needed them. I brought her home here where she just deteriorated rapidly. I begged them for a Macmillan Nurse. I was told I couldn't have one because they were funded for the cancer patients and she wasn't a cancer patient.

All they did was give me a wheelchair to bring her home.

At home, she went downhill rapidly. I got an ex-midwife, who came and sat with her, otherwise I could not leave her. Her arms locked. She was unable to chew and she had trouble swallowing. She had some awful, thick, white dribble continuously pouring out of her mouth. We had to work continuously to keep her clean. I asked for a hospital bed with cot-sides because she was jerking rapidly. She kept falling out of bed. I had to have somebody with her 24 hours a day to stop her falling. I got the hospital bed on the Thursday. She died on the Sunday.

I got a nurse on the Saturday night, and she told me to go to bed, while she sat with her for a few hours. I went upstairs for the first time in 15 days and I slept. The nurse woke me up the following morning. I went down. It was 6.30 am. I tried to wake her up but she would not waken. Her eyes were half-way open, but she was comatose. I got the doctor out. The doctor came at 12 o'clock, and he said she was in a coma, and would not last the night. She died the Sunday at 11.20 am in my arms.

I am extremely bitter. I feel, in myself, that infected meat was to blame, although I cannot prove it and surely the Government should have done something to prove it. She was a beautiful, healthy lady, and there was no reason for her to die.

Harash: What about teeth and fillings or did she have abscesses?

She had quite a few fillings during her life-time but nothing out of the ordinary. There were no other problems with her mouth that I can remember.

Harash: Finally, tell me now about her diet and the type of foods she ate.

She used to eat a lot of junk food. She could not afford the best meat. She was always having mince meat, shepherd's pies, mince and mash, burgers and sausages and she did enjoy liver. She had four kids, so she could only afford cheap meat.

Brian Davies

Brian Davies, an ambulance driver, died at the age of 41 in August 1996 after an illness of eleven months. His wife describes his initial symptoms as having difficulty in walking and balancing and developing shakes similar to those seen in BSE cattle. His symptoms were attributed to muscular pains in his neck. His mental confusion appeared only later. He had diagnosed himself as suffering from mad cow disease. Although his symptoms were typical of Narang disease, his wife was told by doctors he could not have got BSE because he was too old to get BSE. Examination of his brain confirms that he had Narang disease.

We been married about twenty six years and it was in September, 1995 that I first noticed that Brian was becoming a bit withdrawn in himself and generally just a bit down. My sister noticed that as well. Of course, he was out of work and that would always account for some of his depression.

At that time, he was a driving ambulances, helping with the disabled. He had been out of work for many years and had decided to go in and see if he could do anything to help the disabled. He did a six months course and then carried on voluntarily from September onwards. Come the Christmas, Brian was complaining of muscular pains in his arms and his legs and he went to see his GP who said it could be arthritis. A blood test was done and it came back negative but the pain seemed to be getting worse. He took himself off to the Bristol Hospital, the casualty Department. They said his heart and everything was fine and to go back to his G.P.

His doctor said he thought it all stemmed from Brian's neck and that he would arrange for him to be seen by a neurologist. Then Brian's balance started going. This was the January and the appointment wasn't actually until the April. He started losing his balance and. whenever he stood up, he seemed to wobble.

He went to see the doctor again. At that stage, he was going on his own. When he came home, he said: "My balance is all off. I couldn't even touch my nose." He had told the doctor about falling over and the doctor just said: "Not to worry about that.

When you go to see the neurologist he will sort it all out."

Well that was in February. He understood perfectly what was being said. His mental confusion didn't come until later. His balance got worse and it got to the stage where he couldn't go out on his own because he looked as if he was drunk. That was the only way he could describe it himself: as if he was drunk.

My sister bought a flat and Brian wanted to decorate it for her. He wasn't able to because of his lack of balance: he was falling all over the place. He wasn't eating very well.

Everything else seemed fine except, as I said: the balance got worse and I made an appointment for us both to see the doctor. I had to take him because he couldn't have walked outside on his own. This would be February, beginning of March. The doctor was very concerned and told us he'd arrange for a brain scan. He had the brain scan and they did lots of balance tests. By this time Brian couldn't balance on one leg and he couldn't put one foot in front of another. I was just amazed. The scan was clear. There was nothing to be seen to explain Brian's trouble.

At Weston hospital, he was put on a course of vitamin tablets for two weeks and we had to wait for another appointment. The next appointment to come through was for him to go to hospital in March. Then they did a lumbar puncture. While we were waiting for ten days for the results, Brian obviously got worse. He just couldn't sleep and just couldn't understand what was wrong. He was really upset and we stayed up all night. I kept asking: "Is your head fuzzy or dizzy." "I don't feel dizzy" he said: "I just feel as though something is not right."

I phoned the doctor in the morning and I asked him to come out and he just said: "Well, what do you want me to do?". I said: "Well I think he should go into hospital and get it sorted out and have some tests done."

He was sent back to Walton. That was a Monday at the end of March and, on the Wednesday, they transferred him to another hospital and he was in there right until the end of April and they just kept doing scans and lumbar punctures.

I noticed a lot of changes in Brian's personality. They told me he was having difficulty remembering things, I realised they were right. At that stage, he was all right at remembering things from away back but almost nothing of what had just happened

Dennis Hogan

Dennis was 58 years old when he died in 1995 after being ill for three months. He had been a Storekeeper in a local warehouse and had always enjoyed good health with no record of significant dental troubles. He had been married, with a family, for some 40 years at the time of his death. Following an unrelated eye accident , his wife became aware that his behaviour was changing and, within weeks, noticed that he was having difficulty holding a cigarette to his mouth because of a tremble in his hand. Initially, these difficulties were related to stress and strain. He had had a hip replacement at this time, and his main concern was to get back home and back to work. But his driving had become erratic and he never was able to return to work. His wife Shirley, who had known him from childhood cared for him, mainly at home, throughout his illness, and she recalls the events leading up to his death. His symptoms are typical of Narang Disease but no post-mortem was performed.

Dennis was always a fit, healthy man and we were married for 40 years. I had known him since I was a child. He had an accident in 1946 and had to have an artificial eye. In 1992 he fell on the tow bar of my snack bar caravan and gouged his good eye. The doctor saw him at 8 'o'clock in the morning and fortunately saved his eye. Now, the thing that thing that worries me is this. If Dennis had CJD lying dormant in him for so many years, what about the other people that they operated on after him using the same instruments? They should trace them back now and see which patients these were. They should put those patients' medical records straight.

Dennis wasn't normally frightened of anything. One of the first thing I noticed in Dennis when all his trouble started, was when he was driving and a fly got in my car. What a fuss he made. I had to stop the car and get this fly out. I said: "Den, don't be so daft. You'd have thought it was a wasp.

Maybe we started having hard words because he'd started swearing at me because I'd laughed at him. He had not done that before. When I think about it now, I was rotten in a lot of ways because I just didn't know how ill he was. I thought he had found another woman and was just ignoring me.

Soon after having that eye operation, things changed. Even the girls I worked with told me: "Shirley I 'm sure Dennis's behaviour is changing. There is something wrong with him". Looking back, with hindsight, I can remember a growing number of times when I would ask him questions and would get an answer to something entirely different. I'd say: "Den, I didn't ask you that". He'd say: "Oh it's my ears. I'll have to have my ears done". He began repeating himself. His doctor also spotted this and would say to him: "Dennis you've told me this once". Well he was never a man who would repeat again. I noticed other daft little things happening about then. He went for his hip replacement. When I went to visit him in the hospital, he was standing at the door and he said to me" "Oh I'll soon be back to normal. In nine weeks I'll be back at work". The doctor told him: "You won't be back at work in nine weeks Dennis". He said: "Oh, I will". Although the doctor said: "No", Dennis, himself,did not realise how ill he was and could not see any reason why he should not be back to work.

I tried to make him, as comfortable as possible. The day I brought him out of hospital, we laughed as he danced about on his crutches. I blame myself for his discharge from the hospital, for not realising how seriously ill he was. He could have had a few more days proper nursing care in the hospital.

After I brought him home from the hospital, daft little things started happening. He started to go down very quick. I could see a change every day. Twice, I took him to have his ears tested. The doctor said there was nothing wrong with his ears. He started getting aggressive with me.The doctors kept saying: "Shirley there's nothing wrong with him, he has just had a major operation." They never saw the things he was doing, how nasty he could be, nasty, and I mean really nasty. That would get me upset, but I knew there was something wrong and I said to my friend: "Anna, there is something the matter with him".

Then, he went to the doctors to ask when he could drive, because he wanted to get back to work. The doctor told him: "If you feel up to it, you can drive your car". We got in the car and, just as we got out, he hit the grass lawn twice, then went a bit further and I said: "Den, what are you doing?" The next thing, we were heading to go straight through the hedge to the other side of the road. I sat absolutely petrified. I said: "Den, let me drive". He said: "No, it's just because I haven't driven for a few weeks". I said: "Den, I go away for seven weeks and when I come back, I don't drive like that". I can imagine now how he felt. He said there was nothing wrong and started swearing. He said: "I will have to get used to it." I said: "Den, I am petrified." His reply was "Look, I won't get out of the third gear".

He drove me about 15 miles to Anna's farm. I cried all the way. I didn't know what to do, because he was just driving so erratically. When we got up to Anna's he just laughed about it and told her: "I've frightened Shirley to death." I was absolutely shaking but he thought it was a joke. I said: "I've never been so frightened. If I hadn't have screamed out, we were going through the hedge.". He just laughed and said: "I'll have to have some practice". So I said: "Get in my car and just go and drive round and round". He went in the big car park. I saw him doing wheelies but he must have thought he was driving all right.

Well, my insurance was due for my car and I said: "Can you fill that in for me, Den?" Well, I kept going out and thinking: "Where is he". When I came back, I looked to see how he had filled in the form, and I said: "Den, I can't send that. Look how you've written my name". Something happened to him all within a few days. His behaviour had completely changed: he was a very different person. I said: "Den, don't you even know how to spell my name?" Well, he laughed, so I thought: "Right, I'm going to go and see the doctor". Of course, he went mad and said: "There's nought bloody well up with me". We had a stand up row about this and that, and I went up to see his doctor and I said: "There's something definitely the matter with Dennis".

By this time I noticed that when I'd give him his dinner he would put his plate on his knee and start gobbling it up fast as he could, as if he was in some sort of big hurry. I'd say: "Den, why are you eating your dinner like that for? Nobody's going to pinch it". He'd look at me and he'd go slow for a minute and then he'd be back eating fast. At the same time, I had noticed that his hands were not steady - he was having difficulty in controlling them. He couldn't get his food to his mouth without dropping it. I said: "Its off-putting, Dennis, you eating like that". Then, if something awful happened, he'd laugh, even if someone got hurt. I'd say "You're wicked: what's happened to you?" If there was something awful on telly, he'd laugh and I'd say: "Den, you don't laugh at that" and he'd say: "That's funny". He was never like that before.

I told him: "I can't take much more of this". We were arguing and fighting, and we had never done that before. He wouldn't let me help him. His doctor came up with the suggestion that he was having a nervous breakdown by worrying about my business, and about getting back to work and by not get good rest. Then suddenly he started walking with his arms up. I would go and put them down and, well, he got really nasty with me over that. So when we went to Anna's farm, I'd say: "Anna, go and put his arm down. I daren't, because he'll play war with me." Now, if someone else did it, he didn't say anything.

From then on, he got worse. I had the decorators in the bungalow. Phil and all these decorators were smoking. Now, Den had stopped smoking when he went in for his operation but he said to me when he saw them: "Shirley, I've got something to tell you. I couldn't stand all them smoking, so I have started smoking." I said: "Well if you want to smoke, then smoke." Phil asked me: "Shirl, what's the matter with him? He asked me for a cigarette and I gave him one. Don't let him come back in here. They've been taking the mickey out of him, because he can't hit his mouth with the cigarette". Then he went round the bungalow and I heard him talking to Phil. I could not believe it, because he had known Phil for a number of years. Phil was up the ladder and Dennis turned round and said: "I know you, you're out to get me". Phil thought, is he the same man?

After that, I took him to an agricultural show where I bought him some cigarettes, just to see what happened, but he couldn't put it on to his lips. Phil was right. He kept going up in spasms. I got him some orange juice and I gave him it, and he couldn't get it into his mouth. So I said: "Here Den, let me give you it." He said: "Everybody's watching me, don't." I said: "Den, I'm not bothered. Doctor told you you are having a breakdown, and you are in the middle of it now. Read my lips. You've got me over things, I'll get you over this." So I got his orange and put a straw in, and I put them in his mouth.

Now, I run a business, but I just couldn't leave him. I had to take him everywhere. I'd say: "Get in the car. Den, you're like a naughty boy. Get in, do as you're told." This went on for three to four weeks. Then, he started losing things, or mislaying them and became increasingly awkward. He'd say: "I've lost my keys." Then, he would spend hours, looking for his keys. Ask him to get into the car, ask him to do something and he'd do completely the opposite. Den would play war. He would stand and look and look. In the end, I used to have to shout and I'd say: "Will you do as you're told. You're like a naughty little lad but, if you were a little lad, I'd smack you." Everybody saw what I was having to put up with, because I took him everywhere with me. I couldn't do anything else. But all the time, our friends thought we were having family arguments.

He'd promised to buy the girl that works with me an ice cream. As soon as he saw her, he remembered his promise, knew he'd promised Joy an ice cream. That's how I knew it wasn't Alzheimer's. He knew, after he lost his speech, what he wanted to say but just couldn't get the words together and that got him mad. Well, Joy went to get her ice cream - he'd given her money - and when she turned round he'd gone. He was standing in the middle of the show field, and all he could say was he wanted to get me a coffee. So Joy says: "Come on then, we'll get Shirley a coffee" and she brought him back.

A friend of mine's mum had a stroke and he came round to see me. He said: "Shirl, don't think I'm being funny, but it seems to me he's having a stroke." The doctor came round, and told him he was having a complete breakdown. He said: "Dennis, I know you don't believe in nerves and things like that, but you are in the middle of it. If I give you these tablets, in six months you'll look back on it and you'll laugh." He gave him Prozac. I honestly thought he was having a breakdown. Then things started to get worse and worse, so doctor came back. He said: "Shirley, you can't go on like this." He took me out into the garden, so that Dennis could not hear us, and told me: "I think he's got a tumour on the brain". I'm ringing doctor at Middlesbrough and I'll ask him to have a look at Dennis." He rang that doctor and then said: "Right Dennis, I'll go down and see if there is a bed." Dennis started to cry. The doctor said: "Look, he can cure that, if it's something on the brain."

After he was admitted to the hospital, I did not want to leave him because he couldn't feed himself. Then he was talking gibberish. He'd get mad, he knew what he wanted to tell you but just could not. They told me that the man in the bed next to him must have upset him. I said: "Look you'll have to get yourself pulled together." Then they told him it was dementia. I was worried in case it was Alzheimer's. Then, they told me it wasn't. He got to the stage where he could hardly walk.

Now, when I think about it, you see on telly how these cows are. That's exactly how Dennis was. Exactly the same things that you see with them is what I saw in Dennis. I couldn't tell you exactly when that was. Before he went into hospital, quite often I had to hold him like a little lad all time. It was from about the beginning of June that that was happening. I daren't let go of him, so you can imagine trying to go out and do your shopping and holding a man like a little lad.

He had a vacant sort of expression in his eyes. Sometimes I used to say to him: "Den what are you looking like that for?" and he'd say: "I'm not". He didn't know what he was doing. In September, he had no co-ordination, he would spill whatever he had in his hand. He just couldn't do it. So I would say: "Have I to feed you?" Now, he didn't like that. He lost every faculty, one by one. The last one to go was his sight. In the end, I used to have to take him to the toilet in the hospital. He was embarrassed: he didn't want me to go in with him at all. But I said: "Den, you'll have to because if you don't, you'll make a mess." Well this day he got in and shut the door behind him and I couldn't get in. I could hear him but he wouldn't open the door. He must have thought he was at the toilet. I got upset and the nurses said: "Don't worry about it." They were marvellous because they'd knew what was the matter with him.

If I had known what was going on from the beginning, I could have understood it better, because I often got annoyed with him for doing these daft things, not knowing that he could not help himself. Then, they transferred him to Whitby. Even at that time, he used to cry and cry so, deep down, within himself, he knew, when I think about it now. I kept saying: "Look Den, you must get better. We won't be able to go to Tenerife if you don't. We won't be able to do that".

Then, I began to think he didn't know me. My friends would say: "Of course he knows you." I'd say: "Are you going to sing with me", and I would start singing to him. I'd say: "Mary, he doesn't know us", because he seemed to be in a trance. I'd say: "Can you sing our song?" and everybody would stand crying. They'd say "Of course, he can sing your song". So I'd say: "Come on then, sing" and he'd go "Aagh, aagh." That was as much as he could make himself do if he tried.

He went into the hospital at the beginning of August and he died on September 16th. I brought him home about 11 days before he died. I was with him 24 hours a day when he was at home. Laid on the bed in front of me and my friend, they came and gave him a lumbar puncture without any anaesthetic. He screamed and then he cried and he said: "You would bloody cry if you had a hole in your back like this!" Now, I've read you're supposed to give them a general anaesthetic.

After this, he stiffened up and became rigid. He looked a hundred years old and he had a horrible look on his face, like when you're scared. The doctor gave him medication to relax him. It was hard for me when I was trying to change him before they put the catheter in. It used to upset him sometimes when the nurses or doctors went to do anything with him and he always seemed better if I was there. Twice the doctor asked me to be with him, but said he wouldn't really know it was me. Then, in the end, he died with pneumonia. The doctors said he didn't want to die. He went seven days and nights without any water. They said you can live without food, but not without water.

It's over a year now since he died and they told me then that a post-mortem could be done. Well, I can understand my daughters feelings. All my family said: "No, dad had suffered enough". I knew that well enough because I had brought him home and nursed him for 14 days and nights. I never went to sleep. I fed him for so long. He became incontinent. The hospital staff were not keen for him leave. I just got him out for a break. How I got the strength, I don't know. If I had to do it again, I would do it. Then the doctor talked me into having a post-mortem. He said: "If you would let them have a post mortem or take part of his brain". I agreed with him.

But what upset me was that, for the post-mortem, he had to be taken back to the hospital. I didn't want him to go. I kept him in here. He didn't even go to the Chapel of Rest. They brought him back after the post mortem and they had him in a black bag in his coffin. He didn't look like Dennis. But for me, it was Dennis laid there. Ever since, I have had nightmares thinking of him and his face and how he'd aged. After they had an EEG, that's when they told us he had dementia. We asked the doctor and he said I can't really tell, but its a form of dementia. Then my daughter asked if it was like Alzheimer's. All this uncertainty is why I think they should tell you and be honest about it.

When I went to bring him out of hospital, at first, they wouldn't let him come out. The nurse said: "Do you know what's the matter with him?" I said: "Yes he's having a breakdown". She said: "Is that what you've been told?" They tried to put me off, they kept saying there wasn't an ambulance. They didn't think I could manage. The doctors from the hospital came to see me and said they admired me and I said: I want him home. Then he came home and he looked so miserable.

Harash: What did the nurse tell you was wrong with him?

They weren't allowed to tell me. They just said: "That's what you've been told." I couldn't get any answers. Then my doctor told me: "Shirley, I have to talk to you. He has got Creutzfeldt-Jakob disease." So I said what is that? Then he told me "It is same as mad cow disease."

A doctor came to talk to me from Edinburgh and he took some blood while Dennis was alive. He said that was to confirm whether or not he had CJD. We asked the man from Edinburgh and he said: "Yes, that's what it is". The doctor from Edinburgh was in the room with him and saw him going into his spasms and saw how he was. He said there was no doubt about it. He said they'd know better by taking blood from him. But then, they said there was a chance that it could be hereditary. By taking this blood they would know this for sure. My daughters did not want to know. I did want to know, because I wouldn't like to think that my daughters were going to get anything like that. I'd like to know how he got it but I'm never going to know that now. They have told me he definitely died with CJD. The doctors apologised when they found out they had been wrong to begin with and said they were sorry.

The doctor knew from talking to me that I had been taking him to a farm. He said that, if the tabloids got hold of that, it would be awful and that, "If they printed the story, I could lose everything, especially with my having a snack bar." A lot of them think it was just a burger bar, but it was more than that. I do all home baking and food and it wasn't only my business I could lose. I could lose everything because we had taken a mortgage out on this house, and if I kept quiet I could be in for some compensation from somewhere. But that is a load of bull because nobody wants to know anything about it.

I did cook dinner at home every night: chicken, steak, chops, sausage, casseroles, pastas or anything. We ate more meat when we were younger but not so much recently, because it's now too expensive. Just sliced beef.. roast beef. An odd time he had a hamburger or a hot dog. We had liver more often when we were younger because that's all we could afford. I would boil neck or flap of mutton, or the tail of a cow and I would have to take all the meat out and Dennis would eat the stew.

Harash: What about the condition of his teeth?

They had deteriorated. That was the thing that he thought affected him. He has been scratched by cats. Up on the farm, of course.

As long as I live, I will never get over the trauma and the scar which CJD has caused on my life. I certainly didn't want anything to hurt my daughters at all. It was bad enough them losing their dad. I've lost everything. Life has no meaning for me to go on. It's exactly a year since Dennis died. My eldest daughter worries that people think her dad had "Mad Cow" Disease because they'd tend to put a ticket on us all and think we've all got it. You can imagine how that makes you feel.

Maurice Callaghan

Maurice Callaghan died at the age of 30 from new strain CJD, leaving his wife, Clare. Maurice, an engineer from Belfast, Northern Ireland, who had loved beef and burgers, died in November 1995 after wasting away for eight months. He had been a fit young man who rarely needed to see the doctor, and who would cycle more than 100 miles a week as well as being a keen basketball player. Clare gave birth to their second daughter, Aoife, ten days after Maurice died. Their other daughter, Nathan was three-years-old. Maurice had been Clare's childhood sweetheart. Medical experts advised that the body be buried in a specially-limed grave dug to a depth of nine feet instead of the usual six because of the risk of infection spreading. Grave-diggers were given protective clothing and surgical gloves. An inquest found that Maurice had died of new variant CJD. Clare describes to Harash Narang, how CJD killed her husband.

At the beginning of 1995, Maurice began complaining about a pain in the sole of his feet. He changed his shoes. His feet were still very sore, so he took some pain-killers. In February, he complained that he was not sleeping very well. He became very agitated, and said that his feet were so sore he could not sleep. In time, he became more and more agitated and was sleeping less and less at nights. We put it down to stress at work. He went to see the doctor who gave him pain-killers and beta-blockers to try to calm him down so that he could sleep.

During March, I noticed his speech began to slur. We thought it was caused by the medication he was on. By April, I noticed that he was becoming shaky on his feet when he was walking. I also noticed that when he was carrying tea he would be shaking. I remember one morning seeing him at work carrying a cup of tea down the stairs and saw that his tea was spilling. He was shaking. I said to him, "Look, I will carry that down for you."

Another time, we had gone for a pizza and I told him to stay in the car while I got it. When I came back out, he was standing outside the car and had locked the keys inside. His legs started to shake. It was really bad, it was as if he was nervous. He had said it was like pins and needles.

His speech had become a lot worse. His hands and legs were shaking more. His gait and his manner of walking became more and more unsteady, his speech was worse. He was also beginning to be forgetful. He was tired and exhausted all the time: he had no energy. He had become quite withdrawn. He always had been quiet anyway, but he just did not have the same enthusiasm as he had before. He showed less and less interest in things.

He would just say he was tired. I think he knew something was going on in his body. I think he thought it was stress, thought it may have been a nervous breakdown. His work had become a problem: he was worrying about work.

His short-term memory was starting to go. He forgot the PIN number for his cash card. He was waking out of his sleep, and, one night, changed himself to go to work. He looked at the time and saw it was nine o'clock. I had been out, and when I came back he was ready for work. It was nine o'clock at night. He said: "I'm late for work ". I told him that it was nine o'clock at night, and he said: "Oh right, right, right." Sometimes, if he had been sleeping on the sofa, he would suddenly wake up, look at me and say: "Where's Clare?" I would say: "What do you mean?" I put it down to his just having awaken.

While lying asleep he would suddenly he get shakes. While watching television, he would start shouting at the TV as if it was realistic. I remember saying to him, "Calm down, it is only a TV programme." He was having hallucinations. One night I came in, and he thought someone was in the house because he had heard them upstairs. He thought the 'All Blacks' rugby team were upstairs.

Come May his whole character had changed. He showed less and less interest in things. His co-ordination was going. He would knock things over in the supermarket. He would drive to the left hand side of the road. At the time, I thought he was just having a mental block. We knew something was going wrong, but I put it down to stress, or a nervous breakdown. We had a new car in May, and we noticed that he was driving it to the left hand side of the road. He could not co-ordinate the gears and the clutch. From then on I started to do the driving.

The doctors kept putting it down to problems with his feet. In June, they sent him to the hospital, where they put a plaster of

Paris on his feet to give him an instep. He was very unsteady on his feet. He would always want me around if he was going anywhere, or if he had to talk to anybody. He was not really comfortable unless I was with him.

He was still working as a mechanical engineer at Queen's University in Belfast at the start of June. His boss made an appointment to see the university's doctor and Maurice went to see him. Straight away, the doctor made an appointment with his GP, who did some simple tests and then made an appointment for him with a neurologist. Maurice finished work then.

Our daughter would have been coming up three years. He would say: "I can't manage to carry her" even though I had my own difficulties lifting her because I was pregnant. Many a time she would fall asleep on the sofa and I would carry her upstairs, because he wouldn't be able to carry her up.

He went into hospital in July when he was very unsteady on his feet and needed somebody with him. His short-term memory was a lot worse and he was more confused. Maurice had all the tests done. They were all clear. There was no indication of what might be wrong with him. Sometimes, I would have a half hope because he would say he was a lot better that day than the day before, but then, he would be worst the next day. The hospital let him back out again at the end of August but he became worse quite rapidly. He was badly confused, and then he become incontinent. He then began speaking in a whisper, speaking very softly. We would get very little conversation out of him.

All the tests were repeated again in September and they came back clear. They did lumbar punctures, muscle biopsies, brain scans, EEG. They basically didn't find the characteristic EEG traces that are found in CJD cases. I think that they had some idea of what it was, but they could not see the characteristic features. They wanted to observe him over a longer period.

We said we are going for coffee and we are going to see Harash. It's a strange thing such a unique thing that we are sure and the grief and the emotion ...Yes, well it is still very raw at the moment. Yes, it's just a couple of months, next week it is just coming up to six months now and trying to come to terms with it but it is so new and fresh. I guess it is never easy but time so they say is a great healer. It will help for you to meet other people as well, with the same experience. It's tragic isn't it?

Afterwards, the doctor called us and said that he suspected that it was CJD, and he had had experience of that disease through having worked at the CJD Unit in Edinburgh. It was the doctor and his neurologist who told us it could be CJD. He also told us that there was no cure for it and he didn't have long to live. By that stage I was especially worried because I was pregnant. Somebody from the CJD Unit came to interview us that month. They took blood samples, and we completed their big questionnaire. They went through everything and were particularly interested in what he had been in the habit of eating.

We took Maurice home. By that stage, he was bedridden and I was not getting much response from him. He slept most of the time. He had totally lost his speech. We had nursing care, with nurses coming in four times a day and Maurice remained like that until he was taken into the hospice on November 1st. He died three days later.

I have often wondered whether Maurice may have contracted CJD when he visited abattoirs in 1988 while a student at Queen's University. As part of his course, he studied food engineering and the whole slaughtering process in action. The police have interviewed the other students who went on these trips. They were allowed to use any equipment they wanted while visiting the abattoirs. Maurice had Psoriasis on his elbows which he had the habit of picking. Sometimes, the wound on his arm was open, and he might well have been infected in that way.

Harash: What was the condition of his teeth?

His teeth were fair apart from a gold crown which he got a couple of years before because he kept getting an abscess on one tooth and the dentist decided to take it out.

Confirmation that Maurice had died from CJD did not come until after Christmas because couriers from Belfast refused to take the autopsy material to Edinburgh and we had to wait until somebody from the CJD Unit came to Belfast to take it back themselves. The unit phoned the neurologist, who phoned me to tell me that it was definitely CJD.

Marie

Marie died at the age of 60 in 1992 after an illness of five years. Her initial problems of forgetfulness and walking led to her being seen by her own GP and then being referred to a number of consultants who favoured a diagnosis of CJD. Her husband's inability to care for her adequately at home led to her entering a nursing home where her condition continued to deteriorate. Her daughter Pauline, a nurse, who now tells her story, was told by the GP attending at that nursing home that the symptoms shown by her mother were unlike those of CJD and that, in his opinion, it was more probably Alzheimer's. The post-mortem showed the cause of death as Alzheimer's.

The problems with my mum began in 1987. Until then, she'd been a reasonably fit woman. She lived her own life. In 1987, I was living in the nurses' home doing my training, so I used to come home and see mum at the weekend. We used to go into town for a coffee and that was when I first noticed something going amiss. We'd get on the bus and she couldn't find the right change and she'd be laughing about it and say: "Oh, you know, I'm cracking up, I'm going silly." When she was at home she'd put the wrong things in the fridge, just minor things. I took her to the doctor's and she was put on high doses of steroids. Physically, she really did improve a lot, she came on leaps and bounds she could walk about again. She could do her little jobs, but it was then that I noticed her declining mentally. I noticed a sudden personality change that hadn't been there to begin with and I thought at first that she's got a brain tumour because they'd already done a body scan to look for a tumour. She started having problems with her short term memory, difficulties in signing her name, minor things. She just used to laugh and laugh them off. The kind of thing I noticed would be that, when she put a spoon of sugar in her tea cup, there was as much on the table as in the cup.

She then developed a rash over her hands and her arms and quite gross muscle wasting. The GP referred her to hospital under the mental consultant where various tests were done. The last thing he did was a muscle biopsy and diagnosed her as having Glacamicitosis. He started her on therapy and her mobility improved and the rash eventually disappeared.

Physically she was improving, but mentally she became a lot worse. She had quite bad mood swings, personality changes. She started to get almost paranoid. Things she'd never say about people she started to say. I went to see the GP and she was referred back to the hospital where a CT scan was done. The consultant told us that she'd got Alzheimer's disease and that they were then discontinuing the treatment. All we could do was to take her home and get in touch with a social worker. The social worker then went ahead to sort of refer mum to the psychiatrist to arrange for her to get her into day care — sort of plan for the future as it were, but we didn't really get that far because before she even saw the psychiatrist she started with very bad speech disturbances, stuttering, she couldn't pronounce the words.

She'd be like that for a few days and then seem to improve for a day or two. I felt that this didn't sound like Alzheimer: it was something different. She got to the point at home where dad couldn't cope with her. It was dangerous because of the stairs, she was very paranoid towards him, she went towards him with knives and things, she didn't recognise him. Being in the medical profession, I went to see one of my colleagues, one of the consultants and asked as a favour if he would admit her to give my father a break till we could sort out something for her.

I think the worst thing was the sudden jerky movements that she just developed, strong enough to throw her of a chair into a wall, very strong. These jerks led to her being referred to a neurologist. He called it a myoclonic jerk. They again admitted her and she underwent EEG examinations. Afterwards, he saw the family and said that he didn't think she had Alzheimer, and that it was probably CJD and he was 90% sure, but that, without doing tissue sample tests, he couldn't be 100% sure.

Her eyes didn't seem to focus, it was just a fixed stare. It was a vacant expression, she was looking at something and whatever it was wasn't there. Yes, you could walk in front of her, put your hand in front of her and her expression wouldn't alter. There was nothing we could do, we were told. She would probably have between twelve months to two years to live and we should just take her home and treat the symptoms as they arose.

She was still mobile at this stage and he put her on diazepam to try and control the jerky movements. Shortly after she went home she was seen by a doctor from Edinburgh who did a neurological examination and took blood. He told my father, there and then, that he was certain that she'd got CJD and that there was nothing that could be done.

My father wanted to know what CJD was and had to go back and see her own doctor to find out and was told that, they would have to do a post mortem to confirm it. She was then re-admitted to Springfield with these jerky movements which they couldn't really control, they were getting out of hand.

Because we had never heard of this disease, me and my father went to see the local MP who gave us a booklet about the symptoms. It was really a handbook for carers of this disease and the booklet that they gave us detailed the signs and symptoms. It was just the same as mum was suffering at the time.

She started to deteriorate physically again with these unusual postures. She went into a nursing home and within a month of being in the nursing home she was totally incontinent. She still had the jerking movements but, on top of that, she took epileptic fits which lasted from five minutes to fifteen minutes, full blown fits the were. They were controlled as much as possible with diazepam and again she was bed ridden. Within a couple of months she was totally bed ridden, she'd totally lost all power of speech and I wonder whether or not she could actually see because her eyes wouldn't follow you.

She couldn't walk, she couldn't feed herself, she was in a vegetative state really. The GP at the time who looked after her in the home disputed the diagnosis of CJD because he understood that CJD killed within about three weeks. That had been his grandmother's experienced and that suggested to him that it was Alzheimer's. I got in touch with the Alzheimer Association and asked them to send me some literature on Alzheimer and extra literature about CJD. What they sent on Alzheimer's just didn't tally with anything that mum suffered. It seemed more like CJD.

She then went into long periods of unconsciousness, really shallow respirations, and she'd stay like that for three or four days and then just come round from it. This went on for about twelve months and in the end it was actually sort of bronchial pneumonia that killed her in the end. That was about it really.

After she died, the Coroner's Officer came to say that an Inquest would be required because the neurologist and the GP differed in their diagnoses. They said that the Inquest would be on a certain date, so I asked if the results from Edinburgh had been obtained. They didn't even know that samples had been taken to Edinburgh. So after that, I rang Edinburgh myself and was told that the doctor I'd seen was in Ireland. Samples, however, had been taken and the results would not be known for some time and we would be notified as soon as they became available.

So I rang the Coroner's Officer back and told them they couldn't hold the Inquest until the results available. Without them, you can't possibly determine the cause of death. "Well, we may go ahead and have the Inquest anyway", was his answer. Within a week he rang me back to tell me the Inquest was in two days time, that they'd got the results from Edinburgh by phone. When I went to the Inquest there was only one doctor there. That was the doctor who performed the PM and there was nobody from Edinburgh. The neurologist who had actually diagnosed the CJD wasn't called to the Inquest and they said that the results had been obtained from Edinburgh by phone. I rang Edinburgh again and was told that the results had come through quicker than had been anticipated and had been passed on. Mum, they said: did die of Alzheimer which just happened to mimic CJD to the letter.

Harash: Did they tell you what tests were done in Edinburgh?

No, they didn't. They just said they would take quite a few weeks. Right, the bloke who did the PM who was at the Inquest did say they couldn't distinguish between Alzheimer and CJD. I asked for a copy of the Post Mortem report and I've still got it. I've nursed Alzheimer all my nursing career and you can expect an Alzheimer victim to go 5, 10, 15 years, a gradual deterioration. She just didn't appear like that.

I rang the Alzheimer Association, I didn't tell them who I was, I didn't tell them about my mum. I just said I was doing a project, could they give me some information on Alzheimer in the younger patient. So over the phone, they said you can expect to see a very slow physical decline from short term memory loss, gradually becoming worse. I said well what about the physical symptoms.

She said: "Oh, they might have difficulty in screwing jars." I said: "Well what about strong jerky movements, strong enough to throw somebody into a wall." "Oh, no that's not Alzheimer." We were gearing mum's care towards this long term view. Yes, I get patients in all the time and they are all labelled Alzheimer. We've no clear definition or any reason why but because they come in in a confused state or any sort of dementia, they are automatically Alzheimer, because its an *in vogue* word.

She used to get cold sores. She wore dentures for 20 years, maybe more. She came from a very poor family and they would be living on the cheapest. Even when she had us, the four of us, dad had a nervous breakdown when we were little and he lost his job, so we were very poor as a family.

Basically, we used to eat beefburgers, sausage, breast of lamb, the cheapest cuts of meat to make money go further. She used to go to a market garden so we ate a lot of vegetables to fill you up, you know. Like I say: the cheaper cuts of meat she used to use.

Harash: You said you didn't know what this disease was, did you know what BSE or mad cows disease was?

Yes, but only because of the media. We'd heard of BSE but you know sort of only listened halfheartedly really; because it was something that didn't concern us. What made us think was when we saw the neurologist and he said this CJD and we asked: "Well, what is that? We've never heard of it". He said it was some form of BSE. Of course, my father then went, what are you talking about, how come my mum had got BSE? We were just dumb struck.

Margaret

Margaret died in 1984 after an illness of three months. Her first symptoms were that she became somewhat forgetful and then began to stumble and have trouble walking. Initially diagnosed by her GP as due to a nervous breakdown, she was later referred to hospital as her condition worsened. There, she was finally diagnosed as suffering from CJD. She ate calves brains on toast. Her daughter, Vivian, recalls her mother's illness and the circumstances of her death

It all started off in the summer of 1984. My mother had always been spot on, she always remembered, what we were going to do, where we were going for our holidays, every single thing. My husband and I with the children had been down to Wales to his mother's. We called at my mother's on our way back to Yorkshire. It was half past ten in the morning and she was in her dressing gown. She said: "I've been ringing you all week, where've you been?" I said: I told you we were going for a holiday. I can't remember, she said. That wasn't like my mother.

She was always a very smart woman, always dressed and ready for action. She'd always walk up before 9 o'clock to get a newspaper. On this day, it was a Friday, her oldest sister, Mary, who is still alive, was doing the ironing and I thought, that's strange, you do everything. My mother was having a lot of difficulty sorting out the washing, whose socks are these, whose are these. She couldn't sort them out you know.

I thought this isn't like her. Aunt Mary said she's had terrible diarrhoea. I said I'll nip up and get you some arrowroot. Well, we came back up home up to Yorkshire and in a day or two my sister rung to say there was something wrong with mum. She can't remember things. I said: "Get her to the doctors."

So my father and my sister took her to the doctors. The doctor said: "Oh, she's having a nervous breakdown." I thought that was strange, a nervous breakdown is not what my mother would ever have had. She thoroughly enjoyed worrying about things, she loved having a bit of a worry to work out what was going to happen but she never had a nervous breakdown.

It got worse and worse and worse and that must have been August. She couldn't get in and out of a bath to wash herself and she had always been an immaculately clean woman. She stopped being able to say things: she couldn't remember words. Her memory, her speech was going. Her dexterity was gone and she was a very neat. She used to do a lot of dressmaking, now she couldn't even do the buttons up on her blouse She couldn't remember what order to put her clothes on.

My sister got her back to the doctors and the doctor said: "Oh, she needs a good fortnights holiday to put her right." So my sister brought her up to my house. Within 2 days, it was obvious that things were definitely not right. She was stumbling, she couldn't even walk in a straight line, she had to have somebody help her. She couldn't take herself to the toilet.

She had a glazed look on her face. I took her to the downstairs toilet and said: "There you are mum, I'll leave you to it". Ten minutes later I thought she must have finished by now and she was exactly like a statue sitting where I had left her: she hadn't been to the toilet. She was obviously due because I'd given her drink. So, I dealt with her, I put her on the toilet and I thought, well this isn't right. Her speech virtually gone. She would look round as though she was wasn't seeing what she was looking at, so, she was like you see many people in mental hospitals. I would sit her in front of the television and she'd look in the general direction and that was it.

My father and I would be either side of her, holding her arm and we would make her walk for exercise, because she was eating then with our help but she was getting no exercise at all, so she was beginning to put weight on and she's a slim figure. She couldn't balance. Whenever there was a sudden noise, she would jump, so her hearing was all right and I think remained all right to the end. Right at the very end, however, when she was in hospital, I don't think her eyes opened very much.

So then my own family doctor came out to see her and he said: "Your mother is in a complete catatonic state. She needs hospital treatment straight away". So I said it would be better if she went into hospital in Birmingham where her family was rather than up in Yorkshire where I am. So he made a phone call to her doctor in Birmingham and he was very casual about it all. She was admitted to Hollymore Hospital where she very rapidly became incontinent and she was the only bed patient in this mental hospital, well, on the ward anyway.

They gave her 2 doses of electric shock treatment to bring her speech back. Well the first one didn't work so the second one wasn't likely to. So they then said she needs further tests we'll send her to the medical neurosurgical where they did a brain scan. Now this was about the middle of September. She was admitted to hospital on the first Tuesday of September.

When she was in neurosurgical they gave her a brain scan and they took my sister into the room and told her her mother had a virus, an incurable virus. She should be dead by the end of the week if she continues to deteriorate at this rate. But she didn't. She reached a plateau and didn't go really downhill until nearer the end. That's what they said: your mother has a virus and when they transferred her back to Hollymore, the Indian doctor, the one who signed her death certificate, said: "Your mother has Creutzfeld-Jakob Disease". The nurse called it Croits Velt Jacob, and, of course, I went straight to the public library and I found a very small entry under Croits Velt Jacob not Creutzfeld-Jakob Disease. But she didn't: she lasted until November 26th.

I went into the office and I said: "If she is going to die anyway, even if pneumonia sets in, please don't resuscitate her. The doctor looked at me as though I was stupid. He said: "Have you got medical training to say that." I said: "No, I'm just well educated thank you very much." It is very difficulty with these kind of things to know what to do for the best and, in those days, you know, people were not so afraid of CJD as nowadays, because there was no BSE.

Do you know, when she died, they sealed her casket as a fire hazard. In the meantime when she was still alive, after we'd had the diagnosis of CJD a man came from the Radcliffe Infirmary, a doctor who took a full history from my sister and me of my mother which lasted about an hour and three quarters.

He was very interested in the fact that my mother had at one time lived on a farm in Canada. It was a dairy farm and it was way back in the 50s and 40s after the war.

After that he wanted to know if she'd ever been to Papua New Guinea and I said no, why. He said: "Well, it's like a disease that the natives get there called kuru", and he left it at that. He was very interested in the fact that she had lived on a farm and wanted to know whether she'd been in contact with sheep. We said: "No", because you don't get sheep in Western Canada in the Prairies. She had nothing to do with sheep really.

My family, my mother's mother and her father in Birmingham had butchers' shops. My Aunt Mary worked in a butcher's shop but it wasn't the family butcher's shop. She never caught anything, although she is getting a bit ga ga now, but that's old age. He then told me about how scientists used scrapie infected sheep's brains, turned it into a serum and injected it into other animals who had died of a similar disease as a direct result.

I said the only thing my mother has ever had to do with brains was when she ate calves brains on toast. Oh, no he wasn't interested in calve's brains on toast. That was in 1984, before we had heard about BSE on the radio. Shortly after that, after she died, the following spring, it would be in 1987, I heard of cattle dying of this BSE and I looked at my husband and said: "That's how mother caught it, those bloody calves' brains she insisted on eating."

More than once when I was a child, I'd say what have you got there mum. "Oh, brains on toast, have some." Well I couldn't. I've never been a great meat eater, I don't like it and I certainly would never eat brains to my knowledge. I don't know if it was on toast I can only imagine she grilled them. It was always very soft, it used to spread on toast. I don't know how she cooked them, I never wanted anything to do with that and the thought of it makes me heave anyway.

I did know that scientists had managed to turn scrapie-infected brains into a serum and passed the disease into other animals. He also mentioned that monkeys had had it because, in the scientific field, they'd given it to them, laboratory monkeys and that they were the nearest things to humans. But he was not interested in the fact that she ate cow brains on toast because, so far as I could see, BSE hadn't been made public.

My mother was born in Boardsly Green, Birmingham. My grandmother was a butcher. She managed butcher's shops for her father. Well, while my grandmother worked there I do know that she used to play with the entrails of rabbits. My grandmother used to sell rabbits at the butchers and she used to gut them. It was before the war in the depression in the 20s. In those days people would use literally anything from the butchers shop. Nothing was wasted and my grandmother used to press her own tongues, she used to make brawn.

I can remember going to my grandmother's when I was child, sometime in the early 50's and seeing a basin on a slab with a saucer on top and a weight on top pressing what could have been either tongue or brawn because my grandmother cooked a lot. All the family used to eat it.

Harash: Did your mother tell you why she liked brains on toast?

Oh she said it was tasty: it was a delicacy.

Harash: Where did she get these brains?

Local butchers. If you went along to the local butchers, they would be able to sell you calves or sheep's brains. She once cut herself at the time I was in the police force and I said to my mother, "Ah, I've been on a first aid course. Apply direct pressure and raise the bleeding limb", that's what the sergeant said. I remember her complaining about the pressure and how much I had kept it in the air.

Harash: What about her teeth?

She had all her own teeth, Yes she had fillings, one gold one and a gold crown. She had had several operations. First, a hysterectomy in 1957, and then a gall bladder operation in 1968. In fact not long before she got this disease that killed her, she had some varicose veins removed at a private hospital in Solely.

Yes, but I still maintain that, with the incubation period for BSE being several years, it's quite possible she caught the disease through eating those calves brains on toast. When I was on the Kilroy programme, I recently heard a member of parliament and somebody from the meat industry saying that CJD was spreading in France but they didn't have BSE. I made the point on the programme, "No, but they do buy our calves"

Mary

Elizabeth's mother, Mary, aged 67 who was an active brilliant dancer and swimmer suddenly lost interest in her activities and withdrew from her social life. She died from CJD in 1992. She lived in Seaham, Sunderland and was the fourth person in the area to die of CJD. Elizabeth recalls her thoughts and experience of looking after her mother and how the disease developed and the problems the family faced before the diagnosis was confirmed. Mary had been a regular blood donor.

About a year before my mother became obviously ill, my stepfather died and in August of the following year, 1991 she moved to a new bungalow. She loved to argue and debate but when it came to choosing things she'd say "Oh Elizabeth you go and pick the telephone for me. I don't know what colour. You go and choose the vertical blinds". It is only with hindsight I don't think she was quite as talkative as she had been.

She withdrew into herself and began to cut herself away from her previous activities. Her dancing friends would ring up and she'd suddenly decide she wasn't going. I would say to her, "Mum why is it that you are not going dancing so much now?" I couldn't get any answer: she just looked at me. It looked like she was going to speak and I had to put the words into her mouth because I said: "Is it because you're in your bungalow now and you're happier?" And she just said: "Happier".

On Remembrance Sunday my younger daughter went up to see her. When she got there, as she told me later, she knocked on the window and said her gran looked that way to the left and that way to right. The upshot of it was she couldn't remember where her house keys were. We put this down to having just moved house. My daughter climbed through the window.

When my mum was in the bedroom looking for something else, my daughter rang me and said: "I don't know what's going on but you'll have to come up".

When I got there my mum was having difficulty with her teeth. I said: "What's wrong". "I don't know where I've put them" she said. Her younger sister came to visit her at the same time. Mum seemed to be preoccupied. It was just as if she was completely wrapped up in her own thoughts. We found her teeth and handed them to her and she she tried to put them in the wrong way round. So I pulled them out and put them the right way. It was all very weird and alarming. Her sister said: "My goodness", and started to speak to her sister patronisingly, about what pretty watches she had. When she did that, it was as though it brought my mum back to herself and she snapped back at her sister, "Don't patronise me, just watch yourself".

At that time, she would be 67. She was a brilliant dancer and swimmer. In 1986, she got her gold medal at Sunderland Leisure Centre. Her co-ordination, physically and mentally, was not affected. She had a fall. One of her friends said: "Look your mum is not going to appreciate me telling you this and bothering you, but I am a little bit worried".

In November, she must have realised something was going wrong for she asked me what I thought it could be. I told her I thought that she was doing too much and tiring herself out. That was my answer. I said: "I think you ought to stop dancing and swimming quite as much, and relax a little bit more and stop going out as much". She said: "I don't go out as much now".

The most striking thing about it all was the expression you could see in her face and eyes — vacant at first, primitive. What I saw in her eyes was what I would never have expected to see in a human being. It was what I would have imagined early man to look like. Very very primitive.

I went up to see her and got the GP to come out. He said that she had an infection in the middle ear. He just prescribed ordinary 10-day antibiotics. Two days into taking the antibiotics she said: "My eyes". There was a flu epidemic on at the time. So he gave her eye drops and said: "Just leave it for the ten days and give the medication a chance to go through her.

I could see that something really extraordinary was happening because she wasn't responding at all. She wouldn't come down to stay with me. I had to go and sleep on her sofa. She was having very disturbed nights and very confused days. I telephoned to the local GP surgery and, on the tenth day, when the tablets were completed I took my mum to see the doctor again.

Just as I was getting her ready to go down to the surgery on that day I was seeing off a health visitor at the gate and when I went back in she'd fallen again and cut her head.

A nurse in the GP's surgery attended to the wound. Her GP asked her short-term and long-term memory questions. She wasn't using as many verbs and adjectives as she would normally have done. Her sentences were very short. Not necessarily the wrong words, but I noticed for the first time that she wasn't quite lucid. Anyway, she got the right answers.

The doctor said to me "Is this the same lady I saw a year ago?". He said he would get the same doctor who had seen her that last time in hospital to come to her home to talk to her in her own home environment. By then her actual body language was changing, her hesitation was more pronounced by now, she was taking short steps and hesitating and it was a kind of like that. She was feeling dizzy. She was falling.

The doctor said to me "I don't think it's anything psychiatric at all. The upset of her husband dying suddenly is a red herring. Equally, don't be misled by that into thinking it's nothing to worry about. If it's what I think it is, I'm afraid you're in for a really bad time". He sent her to the RVI Hospital to see a neurologist. She was in the acute ward. The charge nurse was a male nurse. He said: "I'll tell you what I think .. this is just my own opinion. I don't think she should be in here. I think she should be in a psychological unit. I think she is schizophrenic. She has very disturbed nights".

I phoned the doctor. I said I'm a bit worried. When I was in there I would take her to the loo but everything was soaking. It was if they were reluctant to touch her or have any close contact with her body. On 7th January I went into the Royal Infirmary and she wasn't there. They told me they had transferred her to the Cherry Knowle, where she has her own little room.

She was able to speak at that point, because when I was talking to her about some pictures on the wall she could seem to be making replies but what she really was doing at this point was repeating the tail end of my sentence.

The doctor said: "Don't you worry. Tomorrow morning she'll be in Sunderland General and on her records there will be no mention that she stayed the night here".

Anyway, the next morning she was in Sunderland General. She had a lumbar puncture and brain scan. She wasn't in control of her dignity. They fitted her with a saline drip. She was not really speaking very much at all. The last time I heard her speak properly was Christmas Eve and that was in the RVI.

Her sister came in with a box of chocolates. We didn't tell her the name of the chocolates but she said: "Black Magic" and that was right. She never ate them, of course, but that was the last time she saw something that she recognised. That was Christmas Eve. She was looking very very ill. Her weight loss was very noticeable. It was awful. They did give her Diazepam. I looked at the chart and when they gave her that her physical movements were more controlled and she was getting more sleep. And I was thinking, "My God. Surely, by now they have decided what this is". I figured in my own mind that there must have been a reason why they weren't giving her this Diazapen earlier just in case it masked any symptoms.

I said: "Can you tell me what's going on?". A young doctor, wrote on a piece of paper "CJD" and I said: "What on earth is that?" That was the very first time I ever heard that term and he didn't want to say anything more.

I'll tell you what she was doing just before Christmas. It was the weirdest thing. She was forever putting her arms in air and holding them up while she walked. One of the sisters said: "I think she thinks she's dancing". She could not put her arms down. When you touched her and put them back down gently, she didn't say a thing about it.

The trembling that I saw was when she was actually lying down. The one jerk I saw and I commented on earlier was when I was in the ward. She was lying flat on the bed and she she suddenly shot up as if she had been catapulted.

I used to read her cards to her. That used to bring a smile to her face. The smile went on all through December and a good part of January. Her smile wasn't real: it didn't mean anything. It was a beaming smile. My mum was there, I was here and my daughter was over here, and I saw my mum track the source of sound from my voice and then when my daughter spoke I saw my mum pick out the source of my daughter's voice. So what she had was flashes of focusing and that gave you hope, false hope. I said to my sister "I'm sure she knew what I saying the other day" but this she did like an antenna, picked up my voice and managed to locate where my daughter was reading at the other side of the room and that is about all she could do.

She became mute. She'd fall and stumble as if she was drunk. All the way through her illness she never questioned anything, was never really aware that she was ill.

The doctor said to me there was someone coming to see me from Edinburgh. He came and he asked me questions about her diet and what she had been in the habit of eating, I think that was on 25th January. He managed to take some blood from her. She died on 11th February.

The most noticeable thing you would see was her frequent, unexpected and, as far as I could tell, uncontrolled jerking movements in her arms and legs although the continual shaking did seem to have been brought under control.

On 10th February, I'd been there in the hospital with her all day and left to go home shortly before 9 o'clock. Within half an hour, there was a phone call from the hospital. She was deteriorating quickly. I went straight back and got there by about quarter past nine. By then, all the tubes were out of her and she was propped up, almost sitting. She was totally still, there was no movement. Whether they had given her a drug or something, I don't know. Her breathing was becoming more and more infrequent till eventually she stopped completely. She'd had no solid food since November, and had to survive on nothing but semi-liquids since then.

While he was alive, her husband did enjoy traditional north countryman's food, and so did she. They enjoyed rump and T-Bone steak and puddings and, only sometimes, sausages. But, after his death, she would eat out more often and, when she was in a hurry, make do with things like beefburgers.

She had been a pretty woman when she was younger and, apart from a haemorrhoid operation in 1980 had fairly good health. After suffering toothache at one stage, she had gone to the Dentist's where all her teeth removed. That was when she was working in the National Coal Board Canteen. She had occasionally been a blood donor, probably only irregularly.

Donald Spears

Donald Spears, a 27 year old man, had been happily married for a few months. When he was about seven, he had the growth hormone treatment between 1976 and 1981. In 1992, he was notified that some patients had become infected and died of CJD as a result of the growth hormone being contaminated. When the first symptoms of the disease appeared some two years later, he was treated initially for a common ear infection. Knowing the warning he had been given about the growth hormone treatment he had received, he reminded his doctor that there could well be something seriously wrong with him and he was re-examined by a neurologist at Great Ormond Street. Although all the usual tests were negative, because of his clinical history of that growth hormone treatment, he was diagnosed as suffering from CJD. While he was still alive, his brother, Peter Spears and Donald's wife asked Harash to do his live urine test and they tell their experience of the disease as it developed over a period of 18 months. Harash carried out this test and was able to confirm that Donald was, in fact, suffering from CJD. It was at this interview that Donald asked Harash:- How long I've got to live?" 18 months after this interview, Donald is still alive but in very poor condition.

Donald, as you can see, is a happy-go-lucky man, fond of joking, joking all the time. He had nothing to worry about. For four or five years, between 1976 and 1981, he had received growth hormone injections. In about 1992 or 1993, we had an official letter, the same general letter that was sent out to everyone who had received that treatment, letting us know that there might well have been something wrong with the growth hormone given to Donald and that it might have been contaminated with CJD virus. He received that letter in 1992 or 1993. I can't remember which. I've got it somewhere and, basically, it said that growth hormone had caused CJD in certain people. Shortly after that, Donald, did in fact go to see doctors at Great Ormond Street to have a check-up and that is where he first met Dr. Anita Harding, the consultant neurologist.

About a year after he got that letter, Donald started showing symptoms that something was going wrong. That would be in either 1993 or 1994, but I can check the date for you. For some time he had been feeling in his mind that there was something wrong with him. I think that would probably be about August or September, 1994. At that initial stage, he had what I can only describe as mood swings and really, to begin with, he was just more hell-bent on going out. He just wanted to go out and get drunk. He was not sleeping very well. He was not watching television as he always done.

He was working at that time and from the September, when it all started, and building up all the time, he was really burning the candle at both ends. He kept going out drinking even more over the Christmas period and that went on for many months and got even worse when he stopped working.

Well, it was about September, 1994 that I first actually noticed him starting to show signs that he was far from well. It wasn't so much a physical thing, but he did complain of feeling dizzy from time to time. To begin with, he had a few odd fallings over, but nothing to worry about, nothing to make you think there was anything seriously wrong. Within a few months, however,by about Christmas 1994 he was showing a lot of mental changes and his behaviour was changing. During January, he developed flu and several colds. He had been to the GP and was just basically told: "You've got a cold." With the dizziness and the growing difficulty he was having in balancing he was having more and more problems riding his motorbike. It was obvious to us that he was seriously ill, but, when he saw his GP again, virtually all his GP said was, "I think you must have an ear infection, or something like that."

He used to ride a bike for a living but, when the trouble started, he would come in and say: "I'm feeling dizzy." He had a lot of time off work around Christmas that year. He was never sick, just generally feeling unwell. I always wondered about that dizziness and the blurred vision he was having at that time. That wasn't all that worried me. There were a couple of occasions when his work took him to a place he'd known for years and he became confused and lost. He suddenly realised: "I don't know how to get out of here". For someone like him,who does that kind of riding around for a living and knows the place well, that was quite frightening. It was about then that he actually fell off his bike, really came off it. He wasn't seriously hurt, but it was enough to scare him. From then on, his symptoms got gradually worse and he became more and more unsteady on his feet.

When he did go somewhere and get lost he would either phone his boss or else just sit for a bit to clear his mind until it all came back to him. To begin with, we weren't too worried. We thought it happens to us all sometimes. It was only when it continued and got no better that we realised it was no temporary problem but was the start of things to come. He had no choice but to give up work about the end of January. On his last day at work he phoned to say: "I'm not very well. I'm coming home." After that, he didn't go back to work. He was never able to.

He went back to see his doctor and was again told that, basically, it was an ear problem, an ear infection, all that kind of thing. Donald told his doctor: "I think there is something more than that wrong with me" and, somewhat reluctantly,the doctor said: "Well I can refer you to a neurologist,but it will take at least a month and probably about six weeks before he'll be able to see you." I have to say he wasn't really very helpful. The only thing we could think of to do was ring Great Ormond Street ourselves and we did that. We told them we were worried because of the warning we had received about the risk of CJD following the growth hormone treatment and the way Donald was behaving. A couple of days later they admitted him in the afternoon.

They did every test, but, in spite of that, came up with no positive result to suggest a diagnosis. I don't know all the tests, but they did brain scans, tests for MS, epilepsy, spinal fluid test, eye tests and co-ordination tests. They did an EEG test using electrodes on his head. Well, they were all negative but for one which showed there might be a problem with his eye. That was at the end of their tests but unfortunately, well, I say unfortunately, again they found nothing that was of any real consequence. In the end, they diagnosed him as CJD by a process of elimination. Yes. He went in in late March, or early April, and it was about the 20th of April that he was actually diagnosed as suffering from CJD. He was then actually told that he had CJD.

Their diagnosis of CJD was not based on tests they, themselves, did but on their knowledge that he had the growth hormone treatment. They knew he had growth hormones. Yes.

Donald knew that he had that treatment and that is why we decided to get in touch again with Great Ormond Street Hospital. It may be that, as soon as he began feeling unwell, he knew he had CJD because he had heard about some patients having died after this same treatment. He knew that it could be CJD. We suspected it: Donald, I think, knew it already.

Harash: What you are trying to tell me is that, although all the tests were negative, it was only when you told the neurologist that he had had growth hormone treatment and they saw his clinical symptoms, they decided it was CJD. That is the irony of it all. You see, if you hadn't told them about him having had the growth hormone treatment, they wouldn't have been able to diagnose it? Has he been for any more tests?

No, basically, from the time he was diagnosed, he had to go up to Great Ormond Street every two or three months, really just to see the consultant. To begin with, it was Dr Harding but, unfortunately, she is now dead and it's a Dr Woods he should be seeing. Obviously, since he has been immobile, we haven't been up to Great Ormond Street. All they would basically do was give him some co-ordination tests and that would be that.

Harash: It's an amazing thing but, in the same hospital, under that same consultant, Anita Harding, there was another patient with similar symptoms. In his case, when even a brain biopsy was done confirmation was withheld. Its amazing how quickly they can label one and not the other. The slightest clue can put them on the right track.

Donald, even after he was diagnosed, was still mobile and, although obviously he couldn't work, he could still ride his bike occasionally for short periods until about the summer of 1995. It was from early autumn, I think, that he really stopped riding his bike. He did have the Land Rover, and he did drive that for a bit, but then, after September, he stopped driving completely.

Harash: Where would he drive the Land Rover?

Just locally, not far. On the road. For a while, he could drive better than he could walk. The last time Donald drove, he was under proper supervision and, even if you were sitting beside him, he would weave quite badly and he'd be going .. ,I mean he was, out of control. He just wasn't very safe, I don't think. No one told or advised us that he should not be driving or gave us any warning.

After June, when he stopped riding his cycle, he started walking using a stick. He needed that stick to steady himself. When he was out walking, he would tend to veer sort of to the right or to the left although meaning to go straight. He's left handed. He managed to walk with the stick by himself, but he really wanted a stick at first because, when he was out or going to pubs, he didn't want folk to think from his weaving about that he was drunk. It was more to show it was because he was having difficulty walking that he had the stick.

Harash: I think that these things do matter in some cases. Let's ask Donald himself what he can tell us. Donald, did your shaking start on one side or the other, did you have pins and needles?

Donald: I haven't had pins and needles at all ... not had that at all ,and no feeling that I was getting hot or cold in one or the other hand and I never lost sensation.

Harash: Why not hold my hand? You've got a very nice grip haven't you. Very tight, very strong. You still have strength in your arms.

Donald: "Y.e.s .... H.o.w. - l-ong - I - g-ot?

Harash: "How much were you drinking, Donald?" Donald merely laughed and shook his head.

Peter: I don't think he's going to tell you, but I can. At the time of the first diagnosis, he was drinking heavily. He would drink 8 or 9 pints of Guiness a night. That was a lot for Donald, because he had never really been a heavy drinker. That sort of began from about September. It started then and he drank constantly, I would say, till about August or September of last year. He drank a lot of red wine, bottles and bottles of red wine.

Harash: How do you manage to look after him at home?

Peter: We have a Home Help twice a day and the nurse comes in regularly to change him and help however she can and we just take it hour by hour, day by day, just as it comes.

Doreen Guy

Doreen Guy, of Seaham, near Sunderland, died at the age of 61 from CJD in 1993. The first symptoms were tiredness followed by balancing and falling over similar to those seen in BSE cattle and in Narang disease. Then, she became forgetful, would scream and she became fidgety. doctors initially said that she was neurotic. In the end, she started forgetting who her husband and daughter were. Doreen, had been doing 'keep fit' twice a week before the illness struck. Her daughter, Margaret, describes how the crippling condition took hold.

Harash: Margaret, can you tell me what happened, starting right from when you noticed the changes and differences in your mother's health.

Margaret: Doreen had been really fit. She was very active, doing 'keep fit' twice a week, regularly swimming, and exercising in the house.

Harash: Since you mentioned the Keep Fit Classes your mother went to, did you know there was another lady who died from CJD who also went to these keep fit classes in 1992 and lived in Seaham as well?

Margaret: No, I didn't know, there was anyone else in Seaham who died of it. My mother started complaining about feeling tired in May 1992. She was so tired it was untrue, she became extremely tired all the time. She would get up in the morning, be up for three hours and, no matter where we were, she would have to come home to sleep. She would jump into bed fully-clothed, and she never did that previously. She would sleep for a couple of hours, get up for another three hours, and then she would go back to bed. It would continue through the night. She couldn't sleep for a full eight hours.

She stopped getting dressed. She would get up, and would not dress until the afternoon, or would only dress if she had to go out. In the August, she came down to London because I was going on holiday and she came down to mine, a week before. That was the time she had difficulty with my stairs specially these ones. She just couldn't get up them. I more or less had to push her. We were walking down to Hammersmith and she used to hold onto the push chair while walking. She was having difficulty with balance. She used to get dizzy. She would say: " I got dizzy I couldn't even go out of the house". She was having difficulty with balance. We put it down to her being tired then because she was always complaining about tiredness.

A month later, about the middle of September, she was still walking but she was falling over a lot. She just couldn't balance. After that she started becoming a bit forgetful. She would forget where she had put her purse or her keys. She would scream and shout about it. Her whole character seemed to change. She was no longer the really quiet woman she had been.

I was living in London, and she was in the North. My father also worked in London. She did not live in London because we did not have enough money and property is expensive.She spent her time looking after the house and the dog, and visiting her father. She used to do 'keep fit'. We did not see that much of her at that time, and we just thought she was becoming forgetful.

By September, she was very fidgety. If you said to her to stop fidgeting, she would, but she would soon start doing it again. You would forever be telling her to stop. Sometimes when we were talking to her, she would calm down to an extent. She fell over a few times, because she could not balance.

She would say there were spiders on her, and she would constantly pick them off her clothes. Rashes would also appear. If she scratched herself, it would come up red and last for a couple of hours or so. I do not know whether that was connected.

She had problems with her head, constantly suffering badly from migraines. She used to become dizzy, which we used to put down to her migraines. My mum used to think it was just a bad migraine attack and would say: "I had a really bad migraine attack today. I got dizzy, I couldn't even go out of the house." We took her to the doctors. They said that she was neurotic and that there was nothing wrong with her. She used to phone me and say: "Oh, they just tell me there is nothing wrong."

We tried to arrange an appointment with a specialist, but they said we had to wait three months to get an appointment to see a specialist in the Sunderland General hospital. She was just a bit forgetful by that stage. Losing things and forgetting where she had put them. In the end, we went private and paid for a specialist to see her in October.

Up until October, we did not realise that there was anything seriously wrong. We thought she was going a bit crazy. It was frustrating and quite annoying for us, thinking she was not using her head. We would either just say she was being silly, or we would end up getting really angry at her.

I think that there is one thing that my father, who looked after her the most, and I really regret. We did not know what was going on. My mum obviously did not know either, so it was not her fault. I think if we had known, we would have been a lot more patient and understanding.

A doctor came to the house, and he did a few tests, such as asking her to touch her nose and legs. He said that she had lost 20 per cent of her balance, but we did not accept that. By then, she had deteriorated a lot. She could not lift herself up, and we had to guide her when she walked. She had to use a walking stick. She already had one when I went up in October. When I was up a couple of weeks later, she was only using the stick for a little while because she could not hold it. The change was very slow for most of the time. To tell you the truth, we would either just say she was being silly or we would end up getting really angry at her. Now, if I had known more about her illness,it I would have been a lot more understanding and helpful but, at the time, we just didn't know and no-one told us.

She also went outside in her night-clothes a couple of times. The next-door neighbour had to bring her in. She was becoming a lot more forgetful. She would sometimes forget our names.

One time, when she was down at mine, she fell while coming up the first flight of stairs. I could not lift her, and she could not lift herself. I just had to sit behind her on the stairs and try to push her along. She would shout: "Get off me, leave me alone." I was trying to explain if that I did not push her, she would fall down the stairs. I had to sit and wait until someone came home to lift her up into the bed.

By early December, we knew something was drastically wrong. Her whole personality had changed. At the dinner table, she would not touch her own food, but would pick food off everybody else's plate. She was like a pig, putting anything in her mouth, using her hands to pick up the food.

She started losing her speech, and she would jabber a bit. We were trying to get her to say: "jumper" because she was fidgeting with her jumper, so we were trying to get her to say "jumper" but all she would say was, " J.J.J.J.J-per". You know she just couldn't, but she wasn't like that all the time.She would sometimes say: "La, la, la," or sing: "La, la, la," with some music on television. Her speech was not totally gone. She could talk, but she would start talking gibberish or she would miss words out. She was once trying to sing along with 'Songs of Praise', but her words were all jumbled.

She went into the Newcastle General hospital, where they carried out tests for three days over the new year. She stayed there for two weeks... She had these jerks. They said they did not know what it was, and sent her back home. While she was there, she fell out of bed after someone forgot to put up the bar. They found her on the floor. She used to try to get out of bed, becoming a bit agitated. She would scream sometimes, and you would say: "You can't get up, you know I can't lift you." She would try herself, and fall.

We brought her to London in January, and into another hospital. My father worked there, and they said they would see her. At that stage, she could not walk. All of a sudden, she seemed to lose everything. She was incontinent. We had to feed her. It had gone from her pigging out on everything and anything, to it taking us nearly an hour to feed her a small portion of food. She was looking after herself up until over the Christmas and friend would go around and take food and do odd jobs for her.

She could not remember who I was, she could not remember who my father was, she did not know who my children were. She would occasionally get someone's name right. She thought we were in the past tense. She thought that I was her aunt she had last seen years previously. We used to convince ourselves that she was looking at us,but really she was quite vacant. She was just staring around. When we were talking, she would not look. I have been told that she was probably blind.

Then we found out what she had. They had carried out tests on her, including an EEG. They had a suspicion of what it was and what was wrong, and they had flown someone down from Edinburgh. Within a few hours of his arriving, he more or less said what she had. Up until then, we did not have a clue.

He wanted us to complete a questionnaire with about 100 questions such as: did we live near farms, did she eat sausages? He was not with us when we filled it in, we just marked it off. We saw very little of him. The only time he really talked to us was to inform us that it was CJD.

We asked him how she contracted it, but he did not really have an answer. He said that this was why he was doing the survey. He did not even mention anything to do with beef. It was not in the media then, like it is now. The irony is that she was not a big meat-eater. I know it is the luck of the draw, but she ate very little meat, and what she did eat was chicken. She was more a white-meat person than red meat.

Harash: What about the condition of her teeth?

Margaret: Her teeth weren't that bad. She has a couple of false teeth t for years. She probably only had about four or five fillings. She started tampering with her teeth for some years. I remember she used to grind her teeth quite a bit. She use to grind her teeth just grind them together against each other. She had ground them, as you could see, looking at the top. She bit the top of the enamel here, so you could see she didn't grind them right down to nothing. It was just for appearances. She got her false teeth in 1989-1990. Why are you so interested in her teeth?

Harash: In animal experiments, if we damage their teeth with a dental drill and take the crown off, just like you explained, we found that animals fed with contaminated tissues developed the disease with a much shorter incubation period than animals with healthy teeth.

We used to have cats at home. My mum used to feed them tinned cat food. She would have been scratched lots of times, because one of the cats was very wild. Maybe that did it. We always said it had the wild streak in it. Its father was wild. We got her when I was very small,and it died about 13 years ago.

My grandfather, he did lots of things, he used to work on the coal wagon years ago but he did have his own animals as well. He used to keep greyhounds, and he would go to the local butcher's and bring left-over meat to feed the dogs. He used to boil sheeps' heads,but I cannot remember that he used any other animals' heads. I used to hate the smell of it. My mum may well have fed the greyhounds. This was about 24 years ago.

She was diagnosed in February. We took her home and stayed with her. My dad took the time off work, and did everything for her. In the last two months, she was practically a cabbage. We were doing everything for her. She did not know who any of us were by that stage.

She was having to be fed very small amounts and very often. Feeding her became very slow. You would put it in her mouth, she would maybe chew a bit, but we would really have to encourage her to finally swallow after a long time. In the end, we could not get her to eat anything.

She lived for another eight weeks at home, and died in April. She was 61. CJD was put on her death certificate, but no post-mortem was carried out. My father would not allow it, and, at that time we all agreed with him - me and all my brothers. We felt that no one gave a damn when she was alive, so why should we help them when she was dead. It had been like beating your head against a brick wall to get any help from them. Mind you, if I had known then what I know now, had known more about it at the time, I would have been in favour of a post-mortem.

Fonnie Andrews

Ilya Andrews mother died suffering from CJD in Banbury in 1994 at the age 44. She was born in Holland and moved to England 1979. She moved back to Holland in 1986 and back to England in 1992. She started with having funny feelings and, while walking, would bump into people. She had balancing problems and developed jerky movements in her legs, as seen in BSE cows, a typical feature of Narang disease. Her daughter describes to Harash Narang the clinical symptoms as they developed over a period of 18 months and the painful scar that has been left on the family.

She was born in Holland in 1955, but we moved to England in 1979 and lived there for six and half years until we moved back to Holland where my mother remarried and lived near Rotterdam for another 5 years until she moved to Denmark. She lived there for a year and then she moved back to Holland to stay with me for a year and then she returned to England to live. I moved to England in November of 1993 to live with my mother. She was never ill, the only problem she did have.... You know some people just have a rash that comes up from time to time. That was her only trouble. When I joined her in England, she seemed fine. She seemed to have lost some weight, but she'd had some worries and I thought that she might have lost weight because of the stress that she'd been going through.

In January of 1994, she got shingles on her stomach and that really got her down. She lost her job and she started getting very restless at night. At fist, I thought it was a sign of stress and the doctor gave her some diazepam. After that, she got a funny jerk in her left hand and leg and everybody thought it might be because of the medication reacting on her. She stopped the medication but the restless legs kept going on. Nothing would help to stop the jerks in her legs. She couldn't sleep at all.

Sometimes, I would sleep next to her and suddenly she would kick me fairly painful. Going from there, she started to lose her appetite and it happened all so quick. It wasn't as though it was slowly building up. Every day there was a difference. She didn't want to eat very much. She started seeing funny things. If she wanted to drink a glass of milk, she thought it looked rotten, as if there were black spots in it. She began slowly to lose her balance. This all happened basically at the same time. I noticed it getting worse and her balance going. She used to drive a car, but she had to stop because she couldn't even see the clutch. She didn't want to go shopping any more because she used to bump into people. She didn't want that to happen: it made her so embarrassed. She almost had a few accidents, she couldn't see what she was doing anymore. The shaky thing was definitely first the first symptom, that and her balance. She couldn't walk straight either and tended to move over to one side.

I didn't even know BSE existed, I hadn't even heard of CJD. From the first shaking in her left hand, the troubles spread to her eyesight, her not eating food and her balance. They all appeared more or less about the same time. Sometimes, she wouldn't tell me about her losing her balance, maybe she was ashamed of it, maybe she didn't want to worry me, maybe she was conscious that something was going on, but I definitely know that the shakiness, the restless leg shakiness and eating habits were the first three significant things to be seen.

She knew that something was wrong and we both wanted it sorted out. I knew what was going wrong but, obviously, when you are in a distressed state, you might forget one or two things. She started to get forgetful, like she would forget to turn the tap off. I would say: "You've forgotten to turn the tap", of and she would say: "No, I haven't been near there". She wouldn't be able to make a cup of tea for herself because she would spill it and all the time she was getting worse and worse. It was a twitch, you know. I even thought that she might have Parkinson's disease. We kept going to the doctors'. She would hurt herself by doing things. She would forget she'd put food on the stove and it would burn.

On 28th April, she went to the doctors again. By this time, she couldn't cut her own food any more, she couldn't get dressed, she had deteriorated all in one day. We took her to the doctors at 9 o'clock in the morning and she wasn't suppose to go to the hospital until the 11th May, but the doctor referred her to the hospital in Banbury and she saw a neurologist.

He wanted to have mum in hospital for a week just for some tests. That was good for me because we were getting very tired.

Slowly but surely, mum was able to do less and less for herself. We couldn't leave her alone no more and this all came about in the period between the end of February and the 28th April.

She had a cat scan straight away that evening in the Oxford Infirmary. That showed nothing of any significance significance and she stayed in the hospital for the whole weekend. On the Saturday, she had a lumbar puncture and different kinds of blood tests. All of them showed nothing. Some time at the beginning of May, they did an EEG. There was definitely something wrong because the EEG result was not normal. The muscle spasms that she had were so irregular it was quite scary actually sitting there watching her. The consultant, obviously, wasn't quite satisfied with the EEG and wanted another. That seemed to look a lot better, but it wasn't really. It was only because she was very sleepy and that had calmed her down a bit. The first day she was able to walk and she was still able to have a shower with somebody's help, but now it got to the stage where that wasn't possible any more.

She couldn't bear light and she would get very bad headaches. There was a great difference after she had had the lumbar puncture. For three days, the 8th to 11th, she sort of seemed to cheer up a bit, she seemed to be in better spirits, she seemed to be more aware of what she was doing. Everybody thought she was getting better. Suddenly she went down hill drastically.

Before mother went into hospital, we knew that something was wrong, that she could possibly die. I couldn't see her getting any better and I could still see the other things that were wrong. The twitching in her hands grew so severe as to actually lift her out of bed: she would fall out of bed because of it. By this stage, her right hand started to have a tiny twitch and her legs would sometimes twitch as well.

She started to look up at the wall. Her eyes would wander and she would have.... just an empty sort of look. Yes, her eyes would jump up and down and she didn't know why she was doing it. She said: "I like looking at the ceiling." Her character changed totally. She used to be fairly quiet.

Now, according to my father and my Nan she seemed to go back to the way she was when she was a teenager. So far as I could tell, she always remembered us: it wasn't as if she was going senile or anything. It was just that memory loss.

She became very witty, very funny and she didn't want to be on her own at nights any more, so, somebody started staying with her at nights. Everything happened, everything that, you know like the really bad things, seemed to happen in the middle of the night. The convulsions she had were always round about 2 o'clock. They were quite severe, yes, she could no longer shower, she was drastically losing weight, she was beginning to get very skinny, she couldn't eat although she would try, she did have the spirit to keep trying.

We tried to take her out a few times but, after a while, she just couldn't handle it any more. She came to have tunnel vision so she could only see right in front of her. You would talk to her and she would just not respond. It was as if she wasn't there. By this time, they'd already said to me that it was something serious and to keep that at the back of my mind, although they hoped they would find a cure, you know. She couldn't even sit up properly by that stage. She was definitely having trouble with swallowing but she was still drinking. She was in hospital for 3 weeks. We had her transferred to Banbury Hospital because, for obvious reasons, they didn't have enough beds in Oxford. Her words started to slur and when she would try to say something it would be almost too much for her. It was hard work for her to try to say something, for example she tried to say ambulance and it would come out as "am...bul.. l. l .l" she just couldn't finish it.

She still remembered who we were but, when my brother was with her in the ambulance, he said that she was asleep all the way. She was sleeping with her eyes open. I did try to have her sit up and I would sit behind her and hold her but, after a while, it was just impossible. She still spoke at that time, she still would wake up and she was at the Banbury Hospital for 10 days and, in those 10 days, she never ate.

She stopped drinking 7 days before her death and, a week before she died, they put her onto a catheter, a week and a day it was, because she no longer went to the toilet either. We always talked to her, she had a lot of people coming to see her, sometimes we would stand around the bed but she would not be with it. Then somebody would suddenly say something and then, all of a sudden but only for a few seconds, she was awake, she would say something and then she was gone again.

We tried not to have her have the catheter, but we had no choice in this matter because she was just not passing urine. Anyway one night, about 2 o'clock, she got a very big hallucination which I thought at first was all due to the catheter. She started grabbing for it trying to pull it out. That was the biggest hallucination she had, she started screaming, it wasn't a scream, it was a yell. She started signing and it was very strange. It was as if she was scared of something. From then on, she never spoke again. I believe that some part of her died that night.

When you would approach her too quickly, she was startled, she was frightened, she was scared. She didn't want any medication at all. Se didn't want it, I mean, if she had been able to she would have liked to have been given the lethal injection, because she wanted to end her life. She didn't want us or herself to suffer any more. On the Friday, she really made a point of it that she did not want any more medication when they gave her it. They gave her diazepam when she had an hallucination or convulsion. She had some medication for the twitch but she didn't want to have it. That was still very clever of her even though she didn't respond to us. She would just absolutely refuse to take medication, she would keep it in her mouth and then, when the nurse was gone, she would spit it out. Maybe that was just me seeing that she didn't want the medication, maybe she just couldn't, I don't know which way it was.

She never woke up no more, she was just there with her eyes open. All she would have was the occasional bed wash and they would turn her over. We would play her music. That was it, there was just nothing left of my mother at all. She wasn't eating, drinking, standing, no nothing and then she started to shut down and she died on the Saturday night of the 4th June. Her changes weren't major over long periods of time: there was a change in her every single day, every single day, it was just so rapid it was unbelievable. That's what happened.

So far as what she liked to eat are concerned, she loved to have a battered beefburger. That was her favourite with some chips. She ate that regularly, maybe once a week. Spaghetti bolognese, lamb chops, she loved lamb chops, pork, she basically ate all kinds of meats, that's what she ate but she wasn't a big eater. She would have meat balls made with mince meat. She wouldn't really eat chicken pies or anything like that. Pork, sometimes, but lamb was definitely another favourite, because she couldn't really afford it, it was just a treat.

You asked about my mother's teeth. She did have fillings but I don't think she had had any severe problems, just fillings now and then. She had cold sores, she definitely had them, and she always had a habit of scratching them. I know she always had rough hands, especially in wintry times, because I have the same problem at the moment.

I have 2 brothers who have always lived with her. One of them is 13 and one is 20.

Harash: When it came out in the press that your mother had died of CJD how did people react to you when they knew about it?

Well, at one time, you did hear comments on the street. You would hear, ha ha, mad cows disease, let's have a laugh. At one time, when I was at college, we had a hygiene test, they were talking about different kinds of food poisoning, different kinds and how illnesses were contracted. I mentioned something about CJD going into humans. Somebody laughed and said: "Ha ha, mad cows disease, we watched that on the telly, what a name". You know people would just generally have a laugh and a joke especially when you link it to humans. You'd think it's a joke. As soon as I said it, they said: "Oh, I didn't mean to offend you", but they are very curious about the disease. I refuse to eat beef any more and they can not understand why I do not eat it. Recently, there was an advert in the paper for a local pub and it says: "Anybody who wants to catch the mad cows disease, come to this pub and have a steak". I mean, that was disgusting. We phoned this pub up and we told him that it was very tactless of him to put it in the paper. He said he didn't realise that there was anybody local who had died of the disease.

Harash: Does the disease cause embarrassment? Do you find that people speak to you about it sympathetically or do they look at you as if you are about to pass it on to them?

To begin with, it was like that. My cousin, she used to like a bit of sensation, she would introduce me to people, "Oh, this is my cousin. You know, her mother died of mad cows disease". For a while, people were a bit put off, they wouldn't really like to talk to me, they got very funny and tried to get on with whatever they were doing and that gave me the kind of feeling that I was..... It's changed now, I've done a lot of talking to people, and I've always made my point.